GETTING THE HEALTH CARE YOU DESERVE

IN AMERICA'S BROKEN HEALTH CARE SYSTEM

LAWRENCE W. LAZARUS, M.D.

GETTING THE HEALTH CARE YOU DESERVE
IN AMERICA'S BROKEN HEALTH CARE SYSTEM
Lawrence W. Lazarus, M.D.

The information contained in this book is not intended to provide medical advice to you and your family. It is suggested that you seek guidance from your personal physician.

ABOUT THE AUTHOR

Lawrence W. Lazarus, M.D., has spent his forty-year career specializing in geriatric medicine and psychiatry. He is a past president of the American Association for Geriatric Psychiatry and a recipient of the National Institutes of Mental Health Geriatric Mental Health Academic Award. He is the proud father of three wonderful adult children. Dr. Lazarus is in private practice in Santa Fe, New Mexico.

ACKNOWLEDGMENTS

I would like to first thank my patients who have shared with me their struggles to obtain the health care they needed in a sometimes challenging and adversarial health care system. They have taught me the importance of being assertive, the value of having a health care advocate and the need to rely on one's own inner strength and resilience to overcome illness.

I wish to thank my mentors, who served as excellent role models during my formative years of training--Doctors Ferdinand Bonan and Jay Fink in Philadelphia, and Doctors Roy Grinker, Jack Weinberg, and Jan Fawcett in Chicago.

I especially want to thank my excellent editor, Barbara Feller-Roth, who helped transform my long-winded sentences into understandable English and helped me to be direct, concise, and organized. I would like to thank my son, Dr. Mark Lazarus, who is completing his medical residency at Scripps, for thoughtfully critiquing the manuscript and readily responding to questions about ensuring patient safety in the hospital. I am also indebted to my daughter, Nicole, and son, David, and my trusted friends, Mariana Geer and Doctor Robert Palombo, for critiquing the manuscript, Marvin Zimmerman, for unraveling the complexities of the health care insurance industry, and my assistants, Charlotte Schaaf and Mary Louise Ellis, for preparing the manuscript for publication by working closely with Shelley Schadowsky at Good Life Guide and Mark Coker at Smashwords. I hope that you, the reader, with the help of this book, will be better prepared to obtain the care you deserve from America's complicated health care system.

CONTENTS

Part IV

INTRODUCTION

What Has Happened to Health Care in America: How This Book Will Help You Get the Best Care Possible

What has happened to the quality of health care in America? What can you and your family do to take more control of and more responsibility for your health care to ensure that you get the best care possible?

As a physician specializing in the care of the elderly for almost forty years, I want to tell you how I tried to help my seventy-five-year-old Aunt Susan, who lives in a small community in Florida. Here are the strategies I've used to get the best care for my aunt. They reveal how important it is to be assertive, and how to take more responsibility for yourself and your family's health care.

My Aunt Susan's partner for twenty years, Nicholas, died after a long struggle with cancer. He compensated for his increasing weakness by becoming domineering and protective and making all the family decisions. Consequently, my aunt became less proficient in managing her affairs. After Nicholas died, she became depressed, and her previous mild memory problem became more apparent.

To save money, Nicholas had changed to a less expensive insurance policy, but Susan's long-term physician was not a contracted provider. My aunt had to find a new primary care physician (pcp), and he had trouble obtaining her medical records.

I flew to Florida to be with her at her first appointment. There were more than fifteen patients in the waiting room. After a three-hour wait, we finally saw Dr. Brown, who looked exhausted, irritable, and impatient. At the end of her twenty-minute appointment, which included a cursory physical examination, Dr. Brown prescribed an antidepressant and a tranquilizer for my aunt's insomnia. I took the initiative to schedule her next appointment and got a referral to a psychiatrist and a neurologist.

After returning home, I e-mailed Dr. Brown and the neurologist and psychiatrist. My two most important questions were: (1) Which of my aunt's three physicians would be "captain of the ship" and take responsibility for coordinating her care? (2) Would she need to move from her own home into an independent or assisted living facility?

I waited three weeks without a reply. Finally, I called the neurologist, who said that my aunt's tests suggested mild Alzheimer's disease. He said he would set up an office appointment to personally discuss her diagnosis and treatment options.

Instead of waiting to meet face-to-face with my aunt, the neurologist called her on the phone to convey the diagnosis and told her to call his office assistant to set up an appointment in a month. His behavior was not unlike an oncologist informing a patient by telephone that she had metastatic cancer.

The neurologist began Aricept, a commonly used drug for Alzheimer's disease. My aunt couldn't tolerate the side effects and stopped taking it.

After several unreturned calls to my aunt's psychiatrist, I e-mailed him the following question: "How would you feel if I was treating your mother in Santa Fe and failed to return your calls?" The psychiatrist called me within hours, apologized, and explained he had increased the dosage of my aunt's antidepressant. I urged him to either refer her to a skilled psychologist, or to see her weekly for psychotherapy in order to help her develop better coping skills to deal with anxiety about her failing memory. In spite of my requests, the psychiatrist continued to see her monthly for half-hour appointments focused mostly on her medications.

Since depression can worsen cognitive functioning, my family arranged to call and visit Aunt Susan frequently, hoping it would improve her overall functioning. Nevertheless, her short-term memory gradually worsened.

What has happened to the quality of health care in America? Why, as a physician, was I having so much difficulty communicating with my aunt's physicians? If they didn't respond to another physician's questions, their patients probably experienced similar frustrations. From a professional perspective, here are some likely reasons my inquiries were ignored.

The trusted, sacred relationship developed over time between patient and physician has been undermined by the frequent intrusion of insurance and managed care companies. A high percentage of every health care dollar goes to the administrators of managed care and insurance companies rather than to physicians and other health care providers. Physicians and their staff spend valuable time obtaining authorizations from insurance companies for diagnostic tests, surgery, and other medical procedures. Some insurance plans require the primary care doctor to fill out prior authorization forms for expensive brand-name medication, and to document that generic medications have been tried and found ineffective. All these insurance-imposed expenses require the harried physician to generate more money to keep up with his/her increasing overhead costs, resulting in pressure to see more patients for shorter periods of time.

Although the United States spends a higher proportion of gross domestic product on health care than any other industrialized nation, some health care experts believe that the quality of health care in the United States, compared with that of other industrialized nations, has continued to decline over the past decade. Because of the recent recession and other factors, an increasing proportion of Americans do not have health insurance, thus overwhelming the public health care system and causing patients to either delay care or give up trying to get it. When medical care is delayed, an illness can reach advanced stages, leading to hospitalization and making recovery more difficult and expensive. It is no wonder that the number-one cause of bankruptcy in the United States is unpaid medical expenses.

Primary care physicians (pcp's), like my aunt's Dr. Brown, are paid by commercial insurance companies and government insurance such as Medicare for time spent with patients. They are not paid for communicating with other physicians and family members involved with a patient's care. So there is a financial disincentive for physicians to spend time communicating with other physicians and family members, which leads to fragmentation rather than coordination of patient care. Under the new health care reform (HCR), however, physicians will be encouraged to coordinate care with other health professionals, and be paid to do so. The HCR, unofficially known as Obamacare and officially known as the Patient Protection and Affordable Care Act (PPACA or simply ACA), is due to begin in January 2014.

The increasing cost paid by companies to insure their employees has led corporations to switch to less expensive health insurance plans, often resulting in reductions, limitations, or exclusion of benefits and placing a higher portion of the cost of insurance onto the employee. Continuity of a patient's care can be seriously disrupted when the patient's physician does not have a contract with the new insurer, leaving the patient the arduous task of finding a new physician. That physician will be unfamiliar with the patient's medical history, which is what happened to my aunt.

Frustration over the desire to provide high-quality care and to be the patient's advocate in an adversarial health care system, has contributed to many physicians' early retirement and/or a career change from a clinical practice of taking care of patients to an administrative position. The office staff interactions with patients often reflect the physician's disenchantment.

The current shortage of pcp's will only worsen in the next several years when increasing numbers of baby boomers retire and because the ACA mandates that, beginning in January 2014, almost all Americans must have health insurance. It is estimated that between 39 million and 55 million currently uninsured Americans will have health insurance by the year 2023.

Another factor contributing to the shortage of pcp's is a medical student's attraction to more lucrative, technologically oriented specialties such as surgery and anesthesiology, rather than to primary care fields such as family practice, pediatrics, and internal medicine.

There is no doubt that you, one of your family members, or friends have experienced problems similar to those of my aunt. The following chapters contain practical advice on how to fill in gaps in your knowledge; be a more proactive, conscientious patient; and find the best health care in an often adversarial health care system.

The new Affordable Care Act (ACA) will fix some, but certainly not the majority, of the health care issues that you and your family face. How can you successfully navigate the complicated health care system to obtain the help that you and your family deserve? Read this book. Its practical suggestions are based on my personal experiences as a physician and on the triumphs and misfortunes of patients and their families struggling with the complexities of today's broken health care system.

Part I of the book simplifies the complexities of the new ACA, more widely known as Obamacare, which will greatly affect the quantity and quality of health care for most Americans. It is considered the most important health care reform since the introduction of Medicare. Part I also provides practical advice about how to choose and use health care insurance as it exists today while awaiting major parts of the ACA to become effective in January 2014. Portions of the ACA that have already taken effect are also discussed.

Part II explains practical strategies to reduce your health care costs and the many legal rights you have as a patient.

Part III explains the importance of assuming more responsibility for your health care and the crucial role of your health care advocate. Your advocate can assist you in overseeing your medical care, interact with your health care providers and insurance company, and provide you with emotional support when needed.

This section also addresses psychological factors that can interfere with your attending to early signs of a medical illness as well as ways to overcome these obstacles. These factors may include simply fear of hearing the worst rather than finding out the facts and addressing them. This section also gives practical advice about finding a qualified primary care physician (pcp) and medical specialist, preparing for your initial consultation with a specialist such as a mental health professional, and finding the best hospital and emergency room. It also gives suggestions about preparing for surgery and discusses what you need to know about medications and strategies for surviving a stay in the hospital.

Part IV explains the value (and sometimes necessity) of getting a second opinion. It also discusses the benefits and risks of alternative (non-traditional) health care and the value of integrating these approaches into your traditional health care.

PART I

1

Understanding the Basics of the Patient Protection and Affordable Care Act (ACA)

I n the year 2000, Americans with no health insurance totaled 13.1 percent of the U.S. population. In 2011, the percentage increased to 15.7 percent (48.6 million Americans). Today, three groups comprise the bulk of the uninsured: foreign-born residents who are not U.S. citizens, young adults (ages nineteen to twenty-five), and low-income families (whose annual income is less than $25,000).

Even those who have health insurance find it too limited, too expensive, and too riddled with exclusions. And it currently lacks coverage for pre-existing illnesses. A medical catastrophe can lead to bankruptcy. Unpaid medical and hospital bills are the number-one cause of bankruptcy in America today.

Enter the Patient Protection and Affordable Care Act (PPACA) or simply the Affordable Care Act (ACA). It's also known as Health Care Reform (HCR). The ACA is aimed at remedying the inefficiencies and shortcomings of our current health care system. You'll see all these terms used in the news media. I use ACA throughout this book.

Under America's current health care system, insurance rates are rising steadily because health care costs are increasing at unsustainable rates. So the uninsured often put off seeking care until their illness is far advanced, at which point expensive hospitalization and/or emergency room visits are required. This scenario could be improved if more Americans had health insurance that covered preventative care, early medical intervention, and pre-existing illnesses.

Another shortcoming of our current health care system is that doctors and hospitals are financially rewarded by the quantity of tests, procedures, and hospitalizations they prescribe. The more they prescribe, the greater the profit, so there are few or no incentives for efficiency in patient outcomes and for controlling costs.

It is ironic that even though the United States spends 16 percent of its gross national product on health care costs (the highest of any industrialized nation) and has the most sophisticated technological equipment and hospitals in the world, the success rates for various illnesses and life expectancy lag behind those of many other industrialized nations. The ultimate success of the Affordable Care Act (ACA) will hinge on whether or not it can transform an industry that currently rewards volume into a health care system that rewards efficiency and excellent results.

The Affordable Care Act

Health insurance and the provision of health care will change dramatically in 2014, when most of the changes resulting from the ACA take effect. The ACA legislation was passed by Congress and signed by President Barack Obama on March 23, 2010. The U.S. Supreme Court affirmed the constitutionality of most of the ACA provisions on June 28, 2012.

How important is this legislation? Historian Robert Dallek commented in the *New York Times* on June 29, 2012, "Historians will compare Obama's Health Care Reform to F.D.R.'s Social Security and Lyndon Johnson's Medicare."

The Supreme Court's 2012 decision permits the many proposed improvements to our health care system to proceed.

And the decision provides clarity to states, employers, and consumers about what is expected to be done by 2014.

Here are the main features of the ACA:

In 2014 almost every American will be expected to have health insurance. Those who do not will pay a penalty on their yearly income tax.

The goal of the ACA is to provide insurance by the year 2022 for the majority of the 48.6 million Americans who had no insurance in 2011. Medicaid (federal- and state-financed insurance for the poor and disabled) will account for the major increase in the number of insured Americans. Medicaid will be gradually and greatly expanded, depending on how many more states eventually decide to go along with the expansion. Currently, only twenty-five states are participating in the expansion of Medicaid. That number is likely to change frequently.

Health insurance exchanges are being created to sell insurance to Americans who don't qualify for government-financed insurance (such as Medicaid, Medicare, and Veteran Administration benefits) or who do not have insurance through their employer or their parents' policy, or who are dissatisfied with their individual commercial policy. The exchanges are electronic marketplaces through which individuals and small businesses can buy insurance. The ACA created two exchanges--one for individuals and another for small businesses.

These insurance exchanges are currently in various stages of development by individual states and insurance companies, often with the help of the federal government. As of May 2013, only twenty-three states and the District of Columbia were building their own health insurance exchanges or were in partnership with the federal government. The federal government will build exchanges for the twenty-seven states that until now have elected not to build their own exchange. These insurance exchanges will offer many different health insurance policies with competitive rates that meet federal and/or state standards, and they will compete for the large pool of the qualified uninsured.

Health insurance exchanges were supposed to start providing information and begin enrolling customers around October 1, 2013; however, according to a June 2013 report from the Government Accountability Office (GAO), state and federal officials expect that the rollout of the exchanges from most states will be delayed past October 1. An estimated 2 million Americans will receive insurance through the small business exchanges and 7 million through the individual exchanges.

Details about Major Provisions of the ACA

One major provision of the ACA is its mandate that, beginning in 2014, most Americans must obtain health insurance or pay a penalty on their yearly income tax. The Supreme Court ruled this mandate constitutional on the grounds that Congress has the right to levy taxes.

The tax penalty per individual for not purchasing insurance will be $95 in the first year (2014) and then will increase steeply in subsequent years: $325 per individual in 2015, and $695 the following year. However, there will be no tax penalty (1) if you are unable to find insurance that costs less than 8 percent of your annual income, (2) if you earn so little that you are not required to file an income tax return, (3) if you are a member of an Indian tribe, or (4) if you are a member of a religious group that opposes health insurance.

A second major provision of the ACA is that Americans, beginning in 2014, will no longer be denied health insurance because of pre-existing medical conditions (and pre-existing medical illnesses will be covered) or be charged higher rates because of poor health. Insurance companies will be required to sell policies to everyone regardless of health status. Currently, in some states, patients with pre-existing conditions can obtain insurance by enrolling in "high risk" insurance pools.

A third major provision of the ACA allows adults under the age of twenty-six to be covered by their parents' insurance. In 2014, adults who are twenty-six or older will have to buy insurance independently if they don't have it through their employer or a government program such as Medicaid, Medicare, or the Veterans Administration (VA). But the cost may be more for young adults than it is today because (1) insurers won't be able to set premiums based on risk, and young healthy adults are among the lowest-risk patients, and (2) because young adults will be part of a large patient pool that includes chronically ill elderly patients, whose health care costs are usually much higher. Adults under the age of thirty may be able to buy less expensive insurance, but the coverage will be less comprehensive.

A fourth major provision of the ACA is that insurance companies will gradually no longer be able to restrict the amount of money they pay out annually on claims (the yearly limit), and will eventually no longer be able to restrict how much they will pay for the treatment of illnesses (the lifetime limit). Eliminating these restrictions (referred to as yearly or lifetime limits, respectively) will be gradual and will greatly benefit patients needing long-term health care for chronic illnesses. Currently, and in the past, some health insurance policies set lifetime limits of $100,000 to $500,000--often insufficient to cover a catastrophic illness.

Expansion of the Medicaid Program

Medicaid is a joint federal- and state-funded program that began in the 1960s to provide health care to the poor and disabled. Even though Medicaid expansion under the ACA will be jointly administered by the federal and state government, in the initial years the federal government will pay 100 percent of the cost of the expansion.

Incentives for states to participate in Medicaid expansion include provision of health insurance to a larger segment of the state's poor and disabled. The insurance will cover preventive care and facilitate earlier medical intervention to treat acute medical problems before they progress to chronic illnesses. Providing health insurance to a larger number of a state's citizens may also reduce the burden and cost of emergency room visits and hospitalizations. Improved overall health status of a state's citizens is believed to increase work productivity and to improve parental care of the young, mental functioning, and life satisfaction.

As of May 2013, only twenty-five states had elected to participate in the Medicaid expansion. States electing not to expand Medicaid are concerned that, over time, they will gradually assume an increasing proportion of the financial burden. States not participating in the expansion will still receive their current Medicaid funding from the federal government to continue the states' current Medicaid program.

The ACA had hoped that all states would expand their existing Medicaid program so that eventually between 17 million and 33 million low-income uninsured Americans (the number of people if all states had elected the expansion) would be covered by Medicaid by the year 2022. The expansion of Medicaid, if all states participated, would account for more than one-third of the overall number of Americans currently without insurance who would now qualify for Medicaid.

Who Is Entitled to Medicaid in 2014?

Beginning in 2014, according to federal guidelines, you may qualify for Medicaid if you earn less than 133 percent of the federal poverty level (which in 2012 meant earning less than about $14,856 per year). Because the Supreme Court ruled that states not participating in the Medicaid expansion can decide whether or not to adopt the new, less restrictive federal eligibility level for Medicaid, many states that have opted out of expansion have chosen to follow their more restrictive eligibility requirements, such as requiring that applicants first be accepted for Social Security's Supplemental Security Income (SSI). And a state not following federal guidelines may arbitrarily set the Medicaid eligibility requirement only for those earning less than $10,000 a year rather than the federal guideline of $14,856 a year. So these states make it difficult for the poor to receive Medicaid.

Many state governors and legislative bodies, especially in states with Republican governors and state legislatures, continue to harbor very negative feelings about the ACA—especially Medicaid expansion--partly because of the eventual costs that states will have to assume at a time when many states are already burdened with huge deficits. So, many of these states decided not to expand their Medicaid program. Therefore, the estimated total number of new Medicaid enrollees, which the president and Congress hoped would add an estimated 17 million to 33 million Americans (if all states opted for the expansion), will be considerably lower. Unfortunately, nearly half of all poor Americans currently without health insurance live in states not participating in the expansion (such as Texas, Florida, Kansas, Alabama, Louisiana, Mississippi, and Georgia), which will leave millions of poor people not eligible for Medicaid.

But individuals living in the same states not expanding Medicaid who have an annual income of more than 133 percent of the poverty level (approximately $14,856) but less than 400 percent of the poverty level (approximately $45,960 per year) may be eligible for a federal tax credit to subsidize the purchase of health insurance through their state's health insurance exchange.

The exclusion of the very poor in states not expanding Medicaid is illustrated by the following. If the breadwinner in a family of four works full time, is paid $14 per hour, and has no other family income (yearly income about $25,000), he or she would be eligible for a federal tax credit to subsidize the purchase of insurance through that state's insurance exchange. But if the same person in the same state (one that is not expanding Medicaid) is paid $6 per hour (yearly income about $10,800), he or she may not be eligible to buy insurance through the exchange and would not even be eligible for Medicaid if that state's restrictive eligibility requirement offered Medicaid only to those earning less than $10,000 a year.

Fortunately, states not expanding their Medicaid program now will have an opportunity to expand their program in future years. The history of Medicaid shows that it took several years for many states to participate when it first began in the 1960s.

Health Insurance Exchanges

You may be eligible for a federal tax credit to subsidize your purchase of insurance independently through your state's insurance exchanges if (1) you earn more than 133 percent of the poverty level (approximately more than $14,856 as of 2012) but less than 400 percent of the poverty level (approximately less than $45,960 as of 2012), and (2) you don't qualify for Medicaid, Medicare, VA benefits, or insurance under your parents' policy and you don't have affordable job-based insurance. Health insurance exchanges began providing information and enrolling consumers in October 2013.

Contrary to earlier expectations that small business employers would have several health insurance plans to choose from in the first year, it's now projected that employers may be able to select only one plan. Employees not satisfied with the plan may be able to purchase insurance through the individual exchanges.

It is projected that each state's exchange for individuals will have at least several insurance companies competing for business, thus keeping premiums affordable. Each insurance company will need to meet federal standards that include coverage for pre-existing illnesses, better preventative care, reasonable copayments, a limit on out-of-pocket costs (estimated to be $6,400 per year for individuals), higher yearly and lifetime benefits, and premiums that do not penalize the chronically ill. These policies are expected to be a considerable improvement over current commercial policies.

Some insurance companies will find it administratively easier to issue you a new policy rather than revise your former policy. If you currently have an individual health insurance policy, you may have received notice in the fall of 2013, canceling your old policy and issuing you a new policy that meets federal guidelines. Consider comparing the new policy with others offered through your state's exchange before making your decision.

In August 2013 the private data analysis firm Avalere Health conducted a study of premiums filed by insurers in eleven states and the District of Columbia. The study revealed that the monthly premium for a twenty-one-year-old buying a mid-range policy (known as a silver plan) will average about $270 per month, but that's before a federal tax credit--based on income for those who qualify--that may bring down the cost for many people. Monthly premiums for a forty-year-old buying a silver plan will average about $550. But the cost is much higher for sixty-year-olds—about $615 per month (federal tax credits may bring down the cost). Silver plans are supposed to cover about 70 percent of expected medical costs.

However, those sixty years and older who purchase insurance through a state's exchange could also be the biggest beneficiaries of the tax credit because the credit works by limiting what you pay for insurance to a given percentage of your income.

All these premiums are only estimates based on data from a small number of states. Your premium, if you purchase insurance through the exchange, may vary widely depending on several factors, including what state and region of the country you live in, as well as past medical costs for persons living in your state.

The California Model

California, where one in seven residents is currently uninsured, has been a strong supporter of the ACA, expending more time and money than any other state to build its insurance exchange. The Obama administration hopes that California's exchange, called "Covered California," will be successful and then serve as a model for other states.

In California, insurance rates may rise for some individuals and small businesses. But for others, rates are expected to fall because of federal tax credits for eligible individuals. California is counting on several factors to ensure its success: the ACA's mandate requiring most uninsured Americans to purchase insurance federal tax credits for qualifying individuals and small businesses, and a $236 million federally financed marketing campaign that began in the summer of 2013 to encourage young adults and small business owners to purchase insurance through their exchanges. California hopes to enroll about 1.4 million people through their exchange in 2014 and millions more in subsequent years.

Efforts to Encourage Enrollment

The Obama administration and nonprofit organizations are conducting nationwide efforts to provide information about the ACA and to encourage Americans to enroll in the exchanges, Medicaid, and other insurance options. The ACA authorized funding for facilitators to guide people in making the best choice. In June 2013, a nonprofit group, Enroll America, opened its "Get Covered America" campaign to reach out to an estimated 78 percent of currently uninsured Americans who weren't yet aware of these new insurance options. See www.enrollamerica.org for more information. Health providers, case managers, and health care advocates are also helping people enroll.

What the Insurance Exchanges and Medicaid Expansion Mean to Those with Mental Illness

Many commercial insurance companies pay physicians treating an office patient with a medical illness a high percentage of the insurance's approved fee (often 80 percent), with the patient responsible for the remaining 20 percent. Patients being treated for a mental illness, however, are responsible for between 20 and 50 percent of the approved fee. This disparity often prevents even those with insurance from seeking mental health treatment.

The ACA requires that qualified health plans purchased through insurance exchanges provide mental health and substance abuse treatment at parity (equal coverage) with medical treatment. This means that Americans now living in states where insurance policies provide limited or no coverage for mental illness and substance abuse will finally be able to buy insurance (through exchanges) that hopefully will be equivalent to coverage for medical illnesses. Because the devil is often in the details, it remains to be seen how this will actually work.

The twenty-five states (as of May 2013) that elected to expand their Medicaid program will soon be able to offer Medicaid insurance, which usually pays the entire cost of outpatient and hospital psychiatric treatment for many more Americans with mental illness. Currently, in many states adults can't obtain Medicaid unless they first apply for and are accepted for Supplemental Security Income (SSI), a federal program for the physically and/or mentally disabled. Millions of low-income mentally ill Americans are unable (because of lack of knowledge about the complicated health care system, or their illness, or not having an advocate) or are unwilling (because of shame) to apply for SSI. Fortunately, those states expanding their Medicaid coverage will not require individuals to be accepted into SSI before becoming eligible for Medicaid.

ACA's Impact on Americans with Drug and Alcohol Abuse

Although it's been six decades since medical science concluded that addiction is a disease that can be treated rather than being a character flaw or a sign of moral weakness, only one cent of every health care dollar currently goes toward substance abuse treatment. Only 10 percent of the 23 million Americans with alcohol or drug abuse problems now receive treatment--partly because they deny having a problem, or because of shame and stigma. But a quarter of them (about 6 million) currently do not have insurance, which limits their access to treatment to publicly funded programs that have long waiting lists and are usually run by counselors with limited medical training.

The ACA designates addiction treatment an essential health care benefit for those with Medicaid and most commercial insurance plans purchased through the exchanges. So, starting in October 2013 or soon thereafter, when enrollment begins, and January 2014 when insurance starts, several million Americans with substance abuse problems will become eligible for the expanded Medicaid programs and the insurance exchanges. The number of Americans with substance abuse problems seeking treatment could double, depending on how many take advantage of these insurance plans, and depending on the availability of treatment facilities (which are currently scarce given the expected surge in demand). The number of physicians specialized in treating those with addictions will need to double.

Having insurance can mean the difference between getting into a medically oriented treatment program or waiting indefinitely for publicly subsidized help, as the following demonstrates. Mrs. Ellis' nineteen-year-old son, John, became part of a disturbing trend of suburban teenagers hooked on heroin. Because he was uninsured, he was put on a three-month waiting list for a state-supported hospital program. The family couldn't afford the $28,000 cost of private residential treatment or the $2,000 per month injections of medicine to block heroin's high. Fortunately, because of an early benefit of the ACA that provides insurance under a parents' policy for offspring under age twenty-six, John was able to quickly obtain counseling from a private physician specializing in addiction treatment and also obtain the monthly injections, which, because of his having insurance, now cost $40 per month. He's back in school full time and has a job. Families struggling to help a family member with substance abuse need to take advantage of the opportunities available under the ACA that can open a new avenue for help.

ACA's Impact on Medicare

The ACA has already made some improvements in Medicare. If you were insured by Medicare in 2012, you were already entitled to some preventative care, such as a free annual physical, colorectal-cancer screening, and a modest improvement in your Part D coverage (drug benefits). The following paragraph (you may need to read it several times to understand all the particulars) describes proposed improvements to Part D coverage.

As of 2013, under Part D of Medicare (prescription drug coverage) you pay a monthly premium of $35 and a $250 yearly deductible before Medicare covers 75 percent of drug costs--until Medicare pays out $2,250. You then enter what's termed the "doughnut hole." You are then expected to pay the entire cost of all prescription drugs until your out-of-pocket expenses total $2,930, after which Medicare covers 95 percent of drug costs approved by your Part D plan. If you had Medicare Part D in 2012, you should have received discounts on brand name (expensive) drugs. Over time under the ACA, the doughnut hole will be gradually lowered and then finally eliminated by about the year 2020.

Medicare Advantage (MA) plans (also known as Medicare HMOs), such as United Health and Humana, are for-profit insurance plans that are an alternative to traditional Medicare. The government pays private insurers on a yearly basis depending on the amount of medical care expected to be provided per person enrolled in the particular plan.

Under the ACA, there were supposed to have been reductions in the amount of government monies paid to these private insurers in order to have funds to support other Medicare programs. But in April 2013 the Centers for Medicare and Medicaid Services (CMS) announced that government payments to these insurers would actually be increased. These Advantage plans presently pay for hospital and doctor costs not covered by Medicare Parts A (hospital) and B (doctor visits), and some plans provide extra benefits such as eye care and hearing aids.

To keep up to date about the many ways the ACA affects Medicare, call 1-800-Medicare (1-800-633-4227) or visit www.medicare.gov. You can also obtain the telephone number of your State Health Insurance Assistance Program (SHIP) from the above Internet site. TTY (teletypewriter) users for the deaf and hearing impaired can call 1-877-486-2048. If you need help in a language other than English or Spanish, say "agent" when you call to talk with a customer service representative.

The Eldercare locator, which is a public service of the U.S. Administration on Aging, is an important first step for finding local agencies in every community in the United States. The locator provides information about Medicare-supported home- and community-based services and other Medicare benefits such as transportation, meals, and caregiver support services. Call the Eldercare Program at 1-800-677-1116, or visit the Internet site www.eldercare.gov.

Medicare-Supported Pilot Projects

Pilot projects exploring various payment reforms have already been launched under the Medicare program. For example, Medicare may pay the entire medical team and hospital a set fee for cardiac bypass surgery. Monies are divided among the entire health care team. Medicare hopes to determine whether this payment method facilitates better communication, efficiency, and coordination among team members, which could result in better patient outcomes, shorter hospital stays, and lower costs.

The government is supporting another pilot project called the "medical home," where members of an interdisciplinary team of health professionals work together to provide long-term care in the patient's home. Medicare is studying whether or not early intervention in the home setting can help reduce unnecessary hospitalizations and enhance patient satisfaction by helping patients live as long as possible in their homes.

An Important Medicare Development

There has been a long-standing erroneous belief that for Medicare to continue to pay for care in a skilled nursing facility, for home health or outpatient services such as physical and speech therapy, a patient had to demonstrate "improvement." The Jimmo v. Sebelius case (which began in January 2011) clarified and reaffirmed that Medicare also provides coverage for medically necessary nursing and therapy services if the services are needed to "maintain" an individual's condition or to prevent or slow their deterioration.

So if you feel that you or a loved one was or is presently unfairly denied continued Medicare services because "improvement" was not demonstrated, yet maintenance and prevention of decline has been achieved, you can appeal the denial. Go to Medicare's web site, www.medicareadvocacy.org, to obtain Medicare centers' self-help packets to further understand coverage rules and to contest a Medicare denial for outpatient, home health, or skilled nursing care. The Jimmo settlement applies equally to Medicare Advantage plans and the traditional Medicare program.

Electronic Medical Records

In 2008, about 7 percent of physicians and 9 percent of hospitals used electronic records, but by the end of 2013, more than 40 percent of doctor's offices and 80 percent of hospitals that provide Medicare and Medicaid services will be using electronic records. Doctors and hospitals demonstrating the meaningful use of electronic records receive incentive payments from the federal government.

Electronic records allow doctors and hospitals to receive laboratory and other test results more quickly; they foster teamwork and communication between health professionals; and they track medications prescribed by other physicians to avoid harmful drug interactions and duplicated prescriptions.

The government also provides financial incentives to hospitals and doctors for reporting quality measures and patient outcomes, and for communicating electronically with patients. Safeguards to ensure patient confidentiality continue to be improved.

Americans can take advantage of electronic devices now, such as the Smartphone, to obtain immediate access to past and current medical problems, as the following situation illustrates:

Mr. Samuels, as eighty-six-year-old retired construction worker, had cataract surgery in Los Angeles a month before visiting his son's family in Baltimore. While visiting Baltimore over a long holiday weekend, he developed piercing pain in his right eye. His eye doctor in Los Angeles couldn't be reached and his office was closed. Fortunately, all the information about Mr. Samuels' eye surgery and past medical problems was stored on his Smartphone, so the consulting eye doctor in a local emergency room was able to review the data and quickly diagnose and treat the complication.

Because safeguards to protect confidentiality and security of private medical data on Smartphones and other electronic devices have not been adequately refined, inquire about limitations of your privacy and how best to safeguard it.

The hope is that these and other Medicare-supported projects will clarify what treatment approaches work best for which types of patients. If successful, the best practice models initially studied by Medicare may eventually be adopted nationwide by the health care system and by insurance companies.

Although health care reformers are optimistic about these pilot studies, it could take many years for the results to become widespread policy. Another potential roadblock to adopting best practice treatment models is the part of the ACA that restricts government decision-making from dictating treatment approaches agreed upon between you and your doctor. In other words, the law explicitly prevents these pilot research projects from being used to decide how much and for what specific treatment Medicare will pay, thus protecting decisions made in the doctor-patient relationship. Nevertheless, it is hoped that Medicare-supported pilot studies of the best, most efficient treatments will eventually influence the practice of medicine.

How Improved Medicare Benefits Will Be Paid For

To help pay for the above improvements in Medicare, there will be increased efforts to eliminate waste and fraud. There will also be a reduction in the yearly growth rates of payments to hospitals, other health care facilities, and doctors, with the expectation that they will find ways to economize. In 2013, Medicare payroll taxes will increase by about 3.8 percent for the wealthy (that is, for families with a modified adjusted gross income exceeding $250,000) to help finance improved Medicare services. Improved, more efficient, and more coordinated care will hopefully reduce preventable rehospitalizations and unnecessary duplication of tests, all resulting in reduced Medicare costs.

If You Are Employed by a Large Company

Most large companies (with more than 200 workers), which account for 161 million American workers with insurance, already provide insurance for their employees. Under the ACA, the minority of large companies that currently don't provide insurance, such as big employers in the fast food industry paying low wages, were supposed to provide insurance that meets federal standards and reporting requirements by January 1, 2014, or pay a penalty.

But in early July 2013, the Obama administration announced a one-year delay (until January 1, 2015) for companies to provide insurance for their employees, partly as a concession to big business, but also to allow more time for large companies to better understand and comply with insurance and reporting requirements. The existing insurance coverage of most Americans employed by large companies will not be affected by the one-year delay.

The administration will soon issue clearer guidelines and rules to insurers, employers, self-insuring employers, and others. But large company employers are encouraged (but not mandated) to comply with the law's reporting provision in 2014, as originally mandated.

Under the ACA's provision for states, with help from the federal government, to set up state-based insurance exchanges for coverage for uninsured Americans, tax credits were supposed to be available for qualified lower- and middle-income individuals who were not insured through their employers. But by delaying until January 2015 the mandate for businesses to insure their employees and report their compliance with the ACA, the government may be unable to confirm before 2015 whether or not employers are offering insurance to their employees, making it difficult for the exchanges to know who is entitled to tax credits to help pay for insurance.

By 2015, when large companies not currently providing insurance are mandated to do so, large company employers will choose the insurance plan(s) for their employees. Federal regulations will ensure that the insurance plan(s) meet reasonable standards. If you decide to opt out of your employer's plan, you can consider purchasing insurance from your state's insurance exchange. Consider meeting with a knowledgeable person in your company's human services department. If you're uncertain what is best for you and your family, discuss your options with an insurance agent or a relative or friend familiar with the changing nature of health insurance.

If You Are a Small Business Owner

Starting in January 2015 (because of the administration's one-year delay), if you own a small business with more than fifty employees who work more than thirty hours per week, you are required to offer your employees affordable health care or face a $2,000-per-worker penalty. Depending on the size of your business and the state in which it is located, you may be able to purchase a less expensive small-group policy through a regulated health insurance exchange. If your company has twenty-five or fewer employees, you may be eligible for federal tax credits to help purchase insurance for your workers.

Just a reminder that between now and when these major portions of the ACA come into effect, additional political and big-business pressures may result in further modifications of the ACA. Barely a week goes by without the news media reporting some changes, both large and small, that can affect you and your family. So keep abreast of what is happening both nationally and within your state.

Who Will Provide Treatment?

Family physicians and nurses are currently in short supply. The American Association of American Medical Colleges estimates that in 2015 the United States will have 62,900 fewer doctors than needed. This number will double by the year 2025. By 2020, when most of the remaining uninsured will have health insurance, the American Academy of Family Physicians predicts a shortage of 40,000 family physicians. In 2008 fewer than half of all pcp's were accepting new Medicaid patients. That percentage was higher in 2013, making it difficult for the poor to find care even when they had Medicaid. About one-third of the country's doctors are more than fifty-five years old and nearing retirement.

The aging of the baby boomer generation is another factor increasing the demand for doctors. Medicare officials predict that the number of Americans presently enrolled in Medicare will surge from 50.7 million in 2011 to 73.2 million in 2025 (a 44 percent increase).

The ACA calls for the federal government to fund additional training programs for pcp's in order to provide incentives for doctors in training to enter primary care fields (with special scholarships, and by forgiving loans that students borrowed to pay for medical school). However, the current (2013) crop of first-year medical students won't be ready to enter primary care fields until 2019 to 2021.

Medicaid is expected to provide insurance for about one-third of the newly insured beginning in January 2014. To encourage more pcp's to provide medical care for the newly insured, Medicaid may increase payments to pcp's in 2014 and subsequent years while maintaining or reducing payments to physician specialists and finding other ways to reduce costs.

The ACA will fund the creation of more health care centers based in communities and schools. More clinics will be managed by nurses. There will be increased government support for a National Health Service Corps of pcp's, nurse practitioners, and physician's assistants, many of whom will provide health care to underserved regions (for example, rural regions and Indian reservations) in return for loan forgiveness, medical education scholarships, and other incentives.

Despite all these attempts to provide a sufficient number of health care professionals to meet the exploding demand, there will still be an acute shortage of primary care and other physicians.

Challenges to Successful Implementation of the ACA

1. Not Enough Healthy Americans Will Enroll

According to Jonathan Cohn in the March 27, 2013, edition of the *New Republic*, the success of the ACA, particularly each state's insurance exchange, will depend on a large enrollment of healthy young Americans because their premiums will be needed to offset the larger medical bills of the comparatively smaller number of sick people. If the exchanges don't enroll enough healthy people, insurance companies may eventually need to increase everyone's premiums, thus prompting the healthy to drop out, which could start a vicious cycle. There is also concern that some insurance companies won't participate in the exchanges, thus decreasing competition among insurers, which may lead to higher insurance premiums.

In an attempt to avoid this potential problem, the federal government will provide tax credits to qualified individuals and small businesses. In the summer of 2013, the government, along with support from nonprofit organizations, launched a nationwide education program to encourage Americans to take advantage of the ACA. There are tax penalties for those who are required to purchase insurance but decide not to.

It is hoped that insurance companies offering policies on the exchanges will keep insurance premiums reasonable. In the state of New Mexico, for example, which is participating in both the expansion of Medicaid and setting up its own exchange, insurance premiums are expected to increase only 5 percent in 2014.

2. The Computers and Web Sites Won't Work

The ACA requires the creation of a vast computer network so every state has its own insurance exchange web site. Many states' web sites won't be in operation until after October 1, 2013.

The following is an approximation of how the computer systems will determine what you may qualify for. For individuals applying for Medicaid or insurance through the exchanges, the new computer systems have to first determine whether you're eligible for Medicaid or subsidized private insurance through the exchanges. If you qualify for subsidized private insurance, computers will need to figure out what federal tax credit, if any, you qualify for. To figure out the tax credit, the computer system will need to verify your identity, income, and place of residence, which means communicating with the Internal Revenue Service, the Social Security Administration, and Homeland Security. You'll then be presented with insurance choices from the insurance carriers. Finally, taking the tax credit into account, the system will calculate your premium. The whole online system requires high-level security, given the sensitive nature of the data.

Federal officials are particularly concerned about the many states that have asked the federal government to run their exchanges and web sites. Also, although half the states in the country are currently not participating in the expansion of Medicaid, these states nevertheless insist on determining Medicaid eligibility themselves. Many of these states have restricted eligibility requirements and have a reputation for making Medicaid enrollment difficult.

Because of having to use new computer systems and web sites, states could make it more difficult for low-income individuals to connect to Medicaid web sites, resulting in delays in learning if they qualify. And many applicants who don't have computer skills or access to a computer will need assistance.

5. The Usual Problems Will Be Blamed on the ACA

Some health care experts predict that the first year of the ACA will see the usual problems that occur every year in the health care industry (such as long waits to see a doctor, and insurance companies requiring authorization for expensive treatments), but political opponents will likely exploit even the slightest sign of trouble and blame it on the ACA.

But the most important thing to keep in mind is that starting in January 2014, millions of Americans will get the kind of affordable comprehensive health insurance they never could before. This may happen more slowly in some states than others, but it will be an improvement in the current state of health care in America.

What follows is some practical advice for dealing with the many changes introduced by the ACA and by the shortage of physicians.

What to Do Now About the ACA

Many of the changes to our health care system brought about by the ACA are complicated, so it's more than worth your time to study parts of the law that pertain to you and your family. Discuss your options with a knowledgeable friend in the health care field, a dependable insurance agent, or the manager of your physician's office--people who stay abreast of new insurance options. If you are employed by a large company, make an appointment with an experienced advisor in your company's human services department and learn the benefits and limitations of the insurance policies that are offered. If your company offers only one insurance policy that you find insufficient for your family's needs, look into policies you may be able to purchase through your state's insurance exchange.

If you want to remain under the care of your pcp and physician specialists, find out *now* if they plan to continue accepting your current insurance or the new insurance you are considering come 2014. *Before* selecting a new insurance policy, whether it's Medicare, Medicaid, one provided by your company, or your state's insurance exchange, make certain that your physicians are providers with the insurance plan. Otherwise, you may be disappointed to learn when you call for an appointment in 2014 that you will need to find a new physician that accepts your new insurance.

If you are one of the 7 percent of Americans who have an individual insurance policy, you may have received a notice that your current policy is being cancelled and replaced by a policy with superior benefits mandated by the ACA. Before deciding to accept this new policy, consider comparing it with other policies available through your state's insurance exchange. Discuss your options with someone knowledgeable about the ACA and the insurance industry.

The severe shortage of pcp's will only intensify in 2014 and subsequent years when millions of Americans will gradually obtain insurance. If you do not have a pcp, secure one now for you and your family, even if the first appointment is only to have a physical examination. This may enable you to be included in that physician's roster of patients. If you currently have Medicaid or Medicare or anticipate having this insurance by 2014, find a physician now who is a provider with these government-supported plans because many physicians will not be accepting new patients once their capability to accept new patients is reached.

If you don't qualify for Medicaid or Medicare, or your company does not provide insurance, or you are under age twenty-six but your parents don't have insurance, find insurance through your state's insurance exchange. Choose an insurance plan that best suits you and your family's needs, and see if you may qualify for a government tax credit.

The Obama administration is urging all Americans who need health insurance to report their telephone numbers and e-mail addresses through the government web site www.healthcare.gov so you can be notified of new insurance options. Because many of us do not necessarily know whether we are eligible for Medicaid, the Children's Health Insurance Program, or a tax credit to subsidize the purchase of insurance via the insurance exchange, if you apply for one of these programs, federal and state officials are supposed to be able to check which program you may be eligible for.

2

Making the Best Use of Your Health Insurance Now

T his chapter simplifies the complex, often frustrating world of selecting the best insurance for you and your family, whether from your employer or purchased on your own. It also discusses the ins and outs of Medicare, various strategies to win should your insurance claim be denied, and options you have if you are currently uninsured. I share my personal experiences regarding the advantages of working with an independent insurance agent.

Selecting Employer-Provided Insurance

About 60 percent of insured Americans obtain their insurance through their jobs. Employers (usually larger companies) select insurance plans that are cost effective for the largest number of employees, so the plan may or may not be the best one for you and your family. If you have options (sometimes an employer will offer just one plan), take your time studying the different plans. In general, the more expensive plans provide more extensive coverage. Arrange an appointment with a knowledgeable person in your company's human resources or benefits department to get advice about you and your family's particular needs. The Affordable Care Act (ACA), which begins in 2014, is not expected to cause major changes to the insurance you currently receive from your employer, but it may improve your benefits, as discussed in Chapter 1.

Sometimes an employer (for financial and other reasons) decides to change to another insurance company. The new insurance company may not have a contract with your primary care physician (pcp) or a nearby hospital. So if you have a choice of insurance plans through your employer, investigate whether you can stay on your current plan and thereby keep your current pcp and hospital versus switching to the new plan. If you have to switch, you may have to find a new physician and a different hospital that is contracted with the new plan. It's also helpful to investigate the difference between a high- and low-deductible plan.

Choosing Between a High- and Low-Deductible Plan of Employer-Provided Insurance

As a general rule, the higher the monthly premium you pay, the lower the yearly deductible and co-payment and the lower the total yearly out-of-pocket costs you pay. After these yearly costs are paid, your insurance pays 100 percent of subsequent medical expenses.

High-deductible plans usually specify that the insured may need to pay out of pocket between $1,000 to $20,000 yearly before the insurance company begins paying. These plans are usually best for healthy young people who seldom get sick, don't have a family history of serious illness, and can afford to pay the out-of-pocket costs to meet the deductible. High-deductible plans are usually best for those who simply want coverage for a catastrophic illness or an accident.

Those with chronic illnesses who require many physician visits and medications should consider a plan that has a low yearly deductible (for example, $250 to $500) so the insurance kicks in much sooner (after the deductible is met). Another reason for choosing a low yearly deductible is if you tend to worry a lot about your health or have some intuition about becoming ill, perhaps because family members have had serious illnesses, or you just want peace of mind that you'll be adequately protected, and you have the ability to pay the higher insurance premiums.

Understanding Your Insurance Options

The major types of health insurance are preferred provider organizations (PPOs), health maintenance organizations (HMOs), indemnity plans, and government plans such as Medicare, Medicaid, and Veterans Administration (VA) benefits. Keep in mind that the insurance landscape for some of these plans may change when major portions of the ACA take effect in 2014. The three most popular employer-sponsored plans (PPOs, HMOs, and indemnity plans), which can also be purchased by individuals, are discussed.

As of 2006, PPOs, which are the most popular type---accounting for 40 percent of employer-sponsored plans---encourage you (as the insured) to use the physicians and hospitals that have contracts with the insurance company because costs to the patient are less. Although you can select physicians and hospitals outside the PPO network, the extra cost to you can be very high. The PPO plans tend to be more expensive than health maintenance organization (HMO) plans.

HMOs account for about 33 percent of employer-sponsored plans. Your pcp, whom you select from the roster of doctors in your plan, serves as the gatekeeper and coordinator of all your health care. He or she decides and selects a consultant, if needed. This is another reason for wisely choosing a competent and reliable pcp. If you select doctors or hospitals outside the HMO network, you will be responsible for a large portion of the costs, so check this first with your insurance plan.

Indemnity plans (also known as fee-for-service plans) are the most expensive because you can choose any doctor or hospital without needing a referral from your pcp or approval from the insurance company. After you pay the annual out-of-pocket deductible (which may range from $500 to $2,000 per year), indemnity plans may pay about 80 percent of the cost of services and you pay the other 20 percent. Because these plans are so expensive for both the employer and employee, fewer than 10 percent of employers offer some variation of this plan.

Buying Insurance on Your Own

If you do not have employer-sponsored insurance, are not covered under your parent's insurance, and don't qualify for government insurance such as Medicare, Medicaid, or Veterans Administration benefits, and you can afford to purchase insurance on your own, consider the following factors.

First, you need to be truthful when answering questions on an insurance application. Be honest and disclose any previous illnesses. At the present time, if you do not disclose a previous illness and it recurs, insurance companies can deny payment and cancel your policy. Under the ACA, insurance companies cannot deny coverage for pre-existing illnesses or charge you higher premiums if you have had serious illnesses. So under the ACA, you will not be penalized for being truthful on insurance applications.

If you are purchasing insurance on your own, do a lot of investigation because insurance plans can be riddled with scams. For example, beware of medical discount cards that promise a lot (and usually deliver nothing). These discount cards come up on your Internet screen and are found in magazines and newspapers and/or on television. The cost seems unbelievably low, and you later find out that the actual benefits, if any, are negligible. If it sounds too good to be true, it's usually not true. If you want to check out these discount cards, ask for a list of physicians where you live. When you call the office of these doctors, you'll usually learn that they have never heard of the discount card.

Another type of scam is fake insurance companies that disappear with your premiums. To find out whether or not an insurance company is legitimate and whether there have been complaints lodged against it, contact your state insurance commission to verify that the company in question is licensed in your state. You can go to the National Association of Insurance Commissioners Internet site www.naic.org and check individual companies by clicking on "consumer information source." Then check the Internet site www.ncqa.org to see whether your insurance policy has been accredited by the National Committee for Quality Assurance. After you have determined the legitimacy of an insurance company, google "Consumer Reports: Best Health Insurance" to compare the rankings of insurance plans and to read about consumers' experience with the company.

Another type of insurance to avoid is short-term insurance. It offers six-month policies inexpensively, but there's a catch. If you have to extend the policy for another six months because you want coverage to continue treatment for the same illness, for example, it's like buying a completely new policy. When you go to purchase another six-month policy, it won't cover you for the illness you developed during the first six-month policy. This catch-22 and the scams mentioned above are likely to change under the ACA, so investigate this with a knowledgeable insurance agent.

If you are between jobs and don't have insurance, or if you just graduated from high school or college and don't have a job that provides insurance and you cannot be covered under your parents' policy, the best approach may be to buy regular health insurance and pay the premiums month by month. When you get a job that provides insurance, you simply call the insurance company to cancel the policy and stop paying the monthly premiums for the insurance you purchased. But be sure to obtain proof from your new employer that you truly are insured because some employers have a several-month waiting period before your insurance becomes effective.

Buying Insurance from a Nationally Known Insurance Company or an Independent Agent

Consider enlisting the services of an insurance agent from a nationally known and respected insurance company, or consider the advantages of an independent agent because their income or commission is less influenced by the policy he or she sells you. Independent agents can also provide access to a multitude of insurance companies and plans.

Insurance from a National Insurance Company

Ask the insurance agent to address the following issues so you can make the best decision about which plan to buy. Bring a list of questions with you when you meet with the agent.

1. Compare the financial health of your insurer, making certain that the insurance company has been in business for a minimum of five years. Longer is better because half of new insurance companies fail in the first three years.

2. Is your longtime physician a provider with the insurance company you are considering? If you want to stay under your doctor's care, consider choosing an insurance plan with which your doctor is a provider.

3. Does the insurer provide a variety of plans to choose from? The more choices, the better.

4. Does the insurance plan you are considering have contracts with Board-certified specialists near where you live?

5. Does the insurance company have contracts with nearby hospitals, and are the hospitals accredited by the Joint Commission on Accreditation of Healthcare Organizations (JCAHO)?

Once you have established the credibility of the insurance company, you're ready to study the plans, with the help of the company's insurance agent, that are best suited to you and your family. Find out the particular strengths and weaknesses of each plan. The policies you're considering should have a comprehensive, easy-to-understand summary that provides the following additional information so you can make the best decision.

1. What is not covered as well as what is covered? For example, if you are planning to have a baby, you want a policy that covers obstetric services. Study the fine print of the policy to understand the limits and exclusions of the plan. If you have a family history of heart disease, diabetes, cancer, or other medical problems, make certain that the policy doesn't have severe monetary limits for treatment of these conditions. Under the ACA, beginning January 1, 2014, insurance companies must provide coverage for pre-existing illnesses and supposedly will eventually not have yearly lifetime or illness-related monetary limits. But stay tuned to changes in the requirements expected of insurance companies. The devil is in the details.

2. If you or family members have had one or more serious illnesses in the past, find out if these pre-existing illnesses will be covered by the plan you select in 2013.

3. For insurance policies taken out before or during 2013, find out the lifetime monetary limit that your insurance will pay should you or a family member develop a life-threatening chronic illness. Look for a lifetime maximum of at least $5 million. It's projected that under the ACA, there eventually should be no lifetime maximums, but let's see how this plays out.

4. Review a list of all the brand-name and generic medications that you and your family routinely take and find out whether your insurance plan will pay a good portion of the cost. Calculate your approximate yearly out-of-pocket medication costs.

5. Does the insurance plan cover doctor's office or hospital treatment of mental illness? If you anticipate seeing a mental health provider weekly, you will want to know what your co-payment is (it may vary between $0 and $50 a visit) and whether there is a limit on the number of visits per year that your insurance will cover (sometimes the limit is twenty visits). These restrictions may change under the ACA.

6. Does the insurance plan cover home health care and/or a stay in a nursing home or an assisted living facility? If so, to what extent? It's often necessary to purchase a separate policy for this. The older you are, the more expensive the policy.

7. What specific conditions or injuries does the plan cover for an emergency that may require a trip by ambulance to the emergency room? Should you require an ambulance, it's advisable for you or your health care advocate to notify your insurance company in advance to improve the chances your insurance will pay a portion of the cost. For medical problems that are not life threatening, urgent care centers offer a much less expensive option.

8. At what age will your children no longer be covered by your policy? The cutoff age was previously twenty-one unless your child was in college or graduate school, but the ACA has extended coverage until age twenty-six, and attending school is not required. Many insurance companies have already enacted this change.

Value of an Independent Insurance Agent

If you have a complex legal problem, you need a lawyer. Choosing an insurance policy on your own, whether it's health, life, home, and/or disability insurance, can be confusing and time-consuming. You might want to consult an independent insurance agent.

Because independent agents are not beholden to a single insurance company that pays them a commission, they can search the entire insurance market to obtain the best rates and coverage for you and your family. Independent agents spend considerable time getting to know your family's unique financial and insurance needs. A long-term trusting, beneficial relationship can develop. Some agents meet with you at regular intervals to see whether your changing family needs require changes in your insurance.

To find an independent insurance agent, ask family and friends for a recommendation, consult the Yellow Pages, or google "independent insurance agents" to find one locally. Don't feel obligated to select the first one you meet. Don't be shy about asking the prospective agent about his or her years of experience and training, and get permission to call a few of the agent's clients.

Many agents have initials after their name, such as CEP (certified estate planner), CSA (certified senior advisor), and CLU (chartered life underwriter). Ask what these designations mean and what licensing requirements they maintain. Here are a few examples of the help I received from my independent agent.

Thirty years ago I was paying $1,000 per month for my family's health insurance policy. My independent agent suggested I join the faculty of a nearby hospital, which offered the same benefits for a group policy that covered all the hospital's medical staff and their families. My cost was only $350 per month for the same coverage. There was no charge or commission for his advice.

When I was in my fifties, my agent advised me to take out a long-term nursing and home health care policy. He compared seven insurance companies and recommended the policy I still use today. When I obtained Medicare insurance, he helped me select the best Part D (drug) plan and Medicare supplemental plan.

Four years ago my son was in a graduate school that required students to pay for an inferior medical policy with a lifetime maximum of $50,000. My agent secured an excellent policy that cost $250 a month that supplemented the school's deficient one. My son never became ill, but my wife and I slept more soundly. Even after I moved to a faraway city, my advisor e-mails me yearly for my annual insurance "checkup."

He recently told me about one of his clients, Mr. Weiss, who had an expensive Blue Cross/Blue Shield health insurance policy whose extensive benefits were secure and no longer available on newer policies. A representative from a nationally known insurance company tried to convince Mr. Weiss to change to a different policy with a much lower premium but with substandard benefits. This agent for the "new policy" would earn a 10 percent commission.

Mr. Weiss's independent agent (also my agent) strongly suggested that Mr. Weiss keep the older, expensive policy. Shortly afterward, Mr. Weiss's wife developed an unusual blood cancer that required treatment at the only center in the United States with a specialized seven-month-long treatment program. The treatment was covered by the older policy but would not have been covered by the less expensive one. His agent spent considerable time securing letters from specialists substantiating that his client's insurance company should pay for the expensive, lifesaving treatment. The treatment led to a cure.

Unraveling Medicare

When Americans turn sixty-five, and those younger who have serious disabilities (physical and/or mental), they may be eligible for Medicare.

After a yearly deductible of $250 (which begins every January 1) is paid out of pocket, Part A of Medicare pays for the majority of hospital costs. Part B covers about 80 percent of outpatient medical costs, but currently only about 50 percent of the cost of psychiatric office visits. It is advisable to have a supplemental plan that covers a portion of expenses not covered by Parts A and B and sometimes has extra benefits that cover eye and hearing care.

If you spend time every year in two different locations in the United States and have physicians at both locations, consider choosing a supplemental plan that both physicians have contracts with.

When it comes to psychiatric outpatient services, until major portions of the ACA become effective in 2014, Part B of Medicare covers only about 50 percent of the approved Medicare fee, which discriminates against and discourages the elderly and younger disabled patients from obtaining mental health services. Fortunately, some Medicare supplemental plans cover part of the cost not covered by Part B. The psychiatrist has to be a Medicare-contracted physician for any costs to be paid. It is anticipated that the ACA will gradually end this discrimination and pay 80 percent of outpatient mental health fees, as it does for medical services. In recent years, many psychiatrists and other specialists have ceased being providers with Medicare and Medicaid.

Part D of Medicare (which was added as a benefit in 2006) provides medication coverage. Before choosing a medication plan (there are currently many Part D plans to choose from), make certain that the plan covers the medications you typically need. You can use the formulary finder at the Internet site www.medicare.gov, or ask a knowledgeable pharmacist.

The good news is that since January 2011, because of the ACA, those with Medicare Part D have been paying less for medications because drug makers participating in Medicare agreed to give the government a 50 percent discount on premium drugs and a 14 percent discount on generic drugs. The government passed those savings on to seniors. But the cost to seniors who need expensive drugs is still devastating for those living on a fixed income.

One can easily see that for patients who have Medicare Part D who are taking multiple drugs throughout the year, the amount spent out of pocket can total well over $5,000 a year. For those living solely on Social Security income, drug costs can consume one-third or more of their yearly income. Many seniors needing expensive brand-name drugs have to decide whether to spend their Social Security income on food, shelter, or critically important medications.

There are several strategies you can use to cope with this horrendous situation. For the unmarried person earning less than $12,570 a year, or $16,863 for married couples, there is a special Medicare medication discount program costing $30 a year. Find out about it on the Internet site www.medicare.gov, or call 800-Medicare.

Another strategy is to ask your physician to prescribe generic (if available) rather than much more expensive brand-name drugs. Also, ask if he or she has drug samples of brand medications, sometimes supplied to physicians' offices by pharmaceutical company representatives. (Generic medications are not supplied to physicians' offices.) Here's how this can work:

For many years I have been treating John, an elderly depressed man in the advanced stages of Alzheimer's disease, and also counseling his wife. They live frugally on a fixed income and have Medicare Part D. Because John takes six different medications, he reaches the doughnut hole (see Chapter 1) of his Part D drug coverage by March of every calendar year, after which he has to pay over $5,000 out of pocket.

I have long-standing relationships with sales representatives of several pharmaceutical companies that manufacture some of the medications John needs. I call the pharmaceutical representatives weeks in advance of John's office visit so I have these medications available (which saves John about $5,000 a year). It's gratifying to see the couple's appreciative smiles.

Many large discount stores such a K-Mart, Walmart, and Costco offer as many as 125 different generic drugs for $4 to $10 for a month's supply. You can check out Walmart prices at www.walmart.com. You can also search for Canadian companies that offer large discounts on certain drugs; check the Internet site www.tcds.com. Also, large pharmaceutical companies offer patient assistance programs for persons whose income falls below a certain level. For example, for medications made by Pfizer, you can go to the Internet site www.phahelps.com. Then go to "Assistance Programs," then "Connection To Care"; fill out the form, attach it to your physician's prescription, and follow the directions.

Don't assume that even if you have all three parts of Medicare (Parts A, B, and D), all your expenses will be covered. That is why it is important to consider purchasing a supplemental plan because it pays for some medical costs not covered by other parts of Medicare. But even having all this insurance may be insufficient to cover all your health costs during your twenty-plus years following retirement or if you are an adult on Social Security, Social Security Disability Income (SSI), or Medicare. A recent survey showed that only 25 percent of retirees who had Medicare insurance felt confident in their ability to pay for their medical needs. If you are able, consider setting aside some monies in a savings account to pay for unexpected medical costs, especially because costs continue to increase much faster than inflation. Also consider purchasing--from a highly rated, long-established insurance company--long-term care insurance that pays both nursing home and home health care.

What to Do If You're Without Insurance

In 2005, there were 46 million Americans (about 16 percent of the population) without health insurance. From 2008 until 2011, because of the recession and unemployment (and underemployment), the number of Americans without insurance was significantly higher. A great number of small businesses (about one-third of U.S. employers) don't offer their employees health insurance because they can't afford it. But the ACA, beginning in January 2015, mandates that both big and small employers provide insurance to employees working more than thirty hours per week, or pay a fine.

Of the 46 million Americans without insurance in 2006, about 20 percent got most of their care at the emergency room of their local hospital, yet about 30 percent of these visits were not true emergencies. Also, the uninsured are 50 percent more likely to need hospitalization for what could have been a treatable medical problem (one that does not require hospitalization) if they had insurance and had been able to obtain medical treatment at an early stage of the illness. The current sad state of the uninsured should improve by January 2014, when the ACA mandates that nearly everyone (with financial assistance from the government for low-income individuals) is required to obtain health insurance.

Where the Uninsured Can Get Help Now

Since the 1960s, most states have offered some type of Medicaid insurance (supported by federal and state monies) for low-income residents. Also, the boards of health of many cities and states operate free clinics for the uninsured. In addition, medical school teaching hospitals offer care at fees dependent on the patient's financial status.

You can visit the Internet site for the Department of Health and Human Services, www.hrsa.gov, and click on "Get Health Care." Another useful site is www.insurekidsnow.gov. There is also a nonprofit organization that helps patients resolve insurance, job, and debt problems resulting from illnesses; visit www.patientadvocate.org.

Uninsured patients with mental health problems can likewise contact psychiatric outpatient departments of medical school teaching hospitals, local city and state clinics, and local community mental health centers. Patients with Medicare and/or Medicaid insurance can see private psychiatrists and some psychotherapists who have contracts with these governmental insurances. Also, the National Alliance on Mental Illness (NAMI), which has chapters in most states and cities, publishes a newsletter, supports mental health programs in the community, and helps patients find mental health services. Their Internet site is www.nami.org.

Strategies to Win When an Insurance Claims are Denied

Medical debt caused an astonishing 62 percent of personal bankruptcy filings in 2007, and three-fourths of those Americans filing for bankruptcy had health insurance. The Department of Labor estimates that about one in seven, or 14 percent, of claims under employer health plans (and about the same proportion of Medicare claims) are initially denied, which amounts to about 200 million denials out of 1.4 billion claims per year. It is estimated that one out of four Americans has had a legitimate claim denied by an insurance company.

What is encouraging is that patients who challenged a denied claim were successful in getting the claim paid in more than half the cases. Of those who were successful, more than 90 percent were claims for emergency care that were initially denied (such as a visit to a hospital emergency room). What is especially surprising is that only a small percentage of patients whose insurance claims are denied challenge the denial or go on to appeal it.

Why aren't denied claims challenged? Because of a false belief that the effort won't be worthwhile, not knowing how to fight the denial, or because of apathy and not having the physical and mental strength to challenge the denial. Some patients often don't have a concerned family member or a patient advocate to help fight the battle.

It's best to begin with the simplest ways of correcting the problem. For example, the denial may have stemmed from a simple paperwork error, such as an incorrect diagnosis or treatment code. Have the manager in your physician's office correct the error and re-submit the bill. If the insurance company decided that the medical or surgical procedure was not medically necessary, ask your physician to write a letter substantiating the medical necessity. For example, your doctor could write a letter explaining why a skin lesion had to be removed because of suspected cancer rather than for cosmetic reasons. If you are still recovering from your illness, have a family member or your health care advocate help you challenge the denial.

If you are disputing a denied claim for a hospital bill, first discuss your disagreement with the hospital's billing department and encourage them to dispute the denial with the insurance company. Don't be too hasty to pay the hospital the remaining balance of your bill until you are positive that your primary insurance--and your secondary insurance, if you have it--has paid for all they are responsible for. The hospital has experienced billers and more clout with insurance companies than you have. If you pay the balance of your hospital bill too soon, the hospital billers may be less aggressive in pursuing the insurance company.

If you or your advocate have to challenge a denied claim directly with the insurance company, first have the insurance company give you in writing the detailed reasons for the denial and the written rules for appealing the denial. Try to establish a good relationship with an insurance representative and save his or her name and telephone number. Better yet, talk with the nurse case manager at the insurance company who will likely be more understanding of your clinical issues than the insurance representative. You can also write a detailed letter, including as much supporting documentation as possible, to a specific person who is in charge of denied claims at your insurance company.

If the above steps are not successful and you still think that your claim is justified, consider making a formal appeal. This has become increasingly important because insurance companies have become more aggressive in denying claims, especially for expensive treatments for diseases such as cancer and for chronic medical and psychiatric conditions.

To appeal the denial, if you're insured by your employer's self-funded plan (the real payers of the claims), appeal to your employer's benefits office or human resources department. Try to get all your supporting evidence to the insurance company's medical director because physicians tend to be more clinically oriented and sympathetic than administrators.

If your employer has a contract with a large insurance company and you join the chorus of employees complaining about the insurance company's frequent denial of claims, your employer may consider contracting with another insurance company.

If these steps are not successful, you can contact the Patient Advocate Foundation at 800-532-5274 or check their Internet site, www.patientadvocate.org. This foundation reportedly gets denials reversed (for varying monetary amounts) about 94 percent of the time. You can go to the Internet site for the advocacy group for your illness (for example, cancer) and learn from other patients with an illness similar to yours how they were successful in obtaining payment for a denied claim.

Keep a copy of all correspondence. Throughout the arduous process, exercise patience, politeness, and, most of all, perseverance. Insurance companies know that a high proportion of those appealing denials will give up during what can be a long, drawn-out process.

Another Internet site that can help you with the details of the appeal process is www.patientsarepowerful.org. If you're dealing with a Medicare denial, utilize the Medicare Rights Center at www.medicarerights.org or call 888-466-9050, or call 800-333-4114 to obtain information about the process. If you are appealing a denial by an HMO, call 202-589-1316.

If your appeal is still not successful and you feel that your case is justified, you can take your appeal to your state's department of insurance. For example, Connecticut is among forty-six states with procedures for the independent review of denials. About half of the appeals brought before Connecticut's department of insurance are successful.

Jennifer Jaff directs Advocacy for Patients with Chronic Illness (860-674-1370), www.advocacyforpatients.org. She wins 80 percent of appeals, which makes her conclude that insurance companies are denying claims far too often.

PART II

3

Strategies to Reduce Your Health Care Costs

E mployers turned to less expensive insurance policies for their employees during the economic recession in 2008 to 2011 primarily because of escalating health care costs. These less expensive policies sometimes led to higher deductibles, co-payments that employees had to shoulder, and reduced health care benefits.

It's been estimated that the average insured worker at a large company in 2009 spent $3,826 on insurance premiums and out-of-pocket medical costs, an increase of 9 percent from 2008 (while wages were stagnant).

Health care expenses continue to rise at the rate of 8 to 10 percent a year, and the elderly have greater health care needs, so workers should not assume that medical expenses will be reduced after their retirement. Retirees who rely on Medicare alone to handle their health care expenses and choose not to have a supplemental insurance plan, should expect that Medicare will cover only about half their medical expenses. The amount of out-of-pocket money that retirees with Medicare alone will need to save to pay the other 50 percent of medical expenses continues to rise sharply. For example, the savings that a couple with only Medicare insurance will need for their health care during the twenty-plus post-retirement years was estimated to be $160,000 (per a 2002 study). That figure rose to $240,000 in 2009. So factoring health care costs into long-range financial planning has become a major priority. It is not too early for those in their thirties, forties, and fifties to consider saving money in a special account in case of a medical or other emergency.

There are numerous ways for you, the well-informed consumer of health care, to reduce costs and be proactive in protecting yourself from escalating medical costs. This chapter gives you ways to reduce the high cost of medications and doctor and hospital expenses, become aware of alternatives to an expensive visit to an emergency room, and learn about available options if you lose your job and your insurance. It also discusses the value of flexible savings accounts (FSAs) and health savings accounts (HSAs).

Of course one excellent way of reducing the high cost of medical care (and avoiding doctors and hospitals) is by adopting and adhering to a healthy lifestyle throughout all stages of life. In fact, employers want you to be healthier, which helps them control their health insurance costs. Currently, nearly 90 percent of large firms offer employee programs to stay healthy, such as smoking cessation and weight-control programs. Some companies may even lower your portion of the health insurance premium if you participate in these wellness programs. About 17 percent of big companies currently, or are planning to, impose higher health care premiums on employees who are at a higher risk for impaired health because of smoking and/or obesity. The president of one large U.S. company purposefully built the outdoor parking lot a quarter mile from the headquarters building to emphasize to the employees the importance of daily exercise.

Reducing the High Cost of Medications

Generic medications are much less expensive than brand-name medications. Your physician probably will not know your insurance's particular drug benefits, so before your doctor writes a prescription, ask if a generic is available. Your insurance card usually has the telephone number of its pharmacy department, so you can call to find out the cost of brand-name versus generic medications and whether or not a generic is available. Your insurance card or information booklet may provide a web site that lists prices for generic, brand-name, and alternate but less expensive drugs that have been on the market for a long time and are less expensive yet are often used for the same medical illness. All of these can lower your out-of-pocket costs. You can also compare retail pharmacy prices for specific drugs at the Internet site www.drx.com.

Some pharmaceutical companies offer free supplies of specific brand-name medications for patients whose yearly income is below a certain amount, so it's a good idea to check the company's web site for details. (See Chapter 10 for additional ways to reduce drug costs.)

Ask Your Doctor for a Discount

If you have become uninsured, have a high insurance deductible or co-payment, or are seeing an out-of-network physician, you have nothing to lose by asking your physician to consider your circumstances and request a discount or a payment plan.

If you need surgery, don't be shy about asking your doctor to recommend more than one surgeon and hospital. You can also ask your primary care physician (pcp) what hospital and surgeon he would use if he or she had financial constraints. Also, your insurance company may be able to tell you what various surgeons and hospitals charge in your area.

Weigh carefully the advantages of getting the best care possible given your financial situation. If your financial situation permits, try not to let cost considerations supersede quality. The web site www.hospitalcompare.hhs.gov provides comparative information about a patient's outcome and quality of care.

Before deciding on seeing a specific specialist or having complicated surgery, make sure the physician and hospital are providers with your health plan. If the hospital or the physician are "out of network" (not contracted with your insurance plan), your insurance will pay a much lower percentage of the bill and your financial responsibility could be very high, so check these specifics beforehand with your insurer and/or the hospital's and doctor's billing department.

Most large employers allow you to set aside part of your paycheck (usually between $500 to $5,000 a year) in some type of savings account to pay health care expenses without having to pay income tax on the monies saved for this purpose. This money can be used to cover deductibles, co-pays, prescriptions, and other out-of-pocket medical costs. There are two major types of medical savings accounts: a flexible savings account and a health savings account.

Flexible Savings Account

One type of medical savings plan is called a flexible savings account (FSA). You need to estimate your out-of-pocket expenses for the coming year before you put money into your FSA because if you don't spend all the money for medical and related expenses by year-end (or the first months of the following year, depending on your company's plan), you lose the money that is left over. Determine your annual out-of-pocket expenses for the past few years to arrive at an estimate of your next year's out-of-pocket costs. Underestimate what you put into your FSA for next year's expenses unless you anticipate higher medical expenses. You can sign up for a FSA with your company during open enrollment or after a "life change" (for example, marriage, or the birth of a child). The human resources department at your company may be able to assist you in estimating the amount to put into your FSA.

Health Savings Account

If your family's yearly insurance deductible is higher than $2,300, you may qualify for a health savings account (HSA), which permits you to save pre-tax money for health care costs. It's an alternative to the flexible savings account (FSA). Unlike the FSA, the HSA allows you to keep the money in this account with no time constraints. As long as the money is eventually used for health care expenses, no taxes are paid on contributions into this savings account or on the interest earned. Also, no taxes are required when the money is withdrawn. For the year 2009, a family could have contributed up to $5,950. Some employers help with contributions. Come retirement, you can even spend the money on non-health-related items, although then you'll pay taxes on the money and the interest earned. You can compare different account terms at the Internet site www.vimo.com/hsa. You usually cannot have both a FSA and a HSA.

Alternatives to an Expensive Emergency Room Visit

If you have a minor illness, such as a head cold or the ubiquitous low back pain, rather than going for an expensive visit to a hospital emergency room (ER), it's much less expensive (whether or not you have health insurance) to consider one of the following:

1. Appointment with your pcp.

2. Workplace clinic – Many large companies have inexpensive or no-cost clinics staffed by a nurse practitioner who can handle minor ailments.

3. Large retail chain stores – Many such stores now have clinics managed by nurse practitioners. If your insurance covers these visits, it's far less costly than a visit to an ER.

4. Urgent care clinics – These clinics are for problems more serious than minor ailments. Staffed by physicians and/or nurse practitioners, they are also a lot less costly than an ER visit.

When to Consider the Emergency Room

Hospital emergency rooms are appropriate for serious medical problems, such as signs of a heart attack, a stroke, or a kidney stone. If possible, notify your insurance company in advance of your ER visit and mention whether you will need an ambulance. If you are incapacitated, have a family member or your health care advocate make the call. Otherwise, your insurance company may refuse to pay. Fees for simple visits to an ER can be well over $700 depending on where you live, and use of an ambulance is very expensive. Bring with you to the ER your insurance card(s), an overnight suitcase in case you are admitted to the hospital, a list of medications and the medications themselves, a list of past and current medical problems, and your health care directive. Always keep with you in a safe, secure place your insurance company's twenty-four-hour claims hotline telephone number and the contact information for your health care advocate.

Strategies If You Lose Your Job

If you have the financial means, set aside a cash emergency fund for six months' worth of household, medical, and other expenses if you (or your spouse) were to lose your job. That fund will provide you with some peace of mind if your insurance ends along with unemployment and you incur unexpected expenses. Keep in mind that if your insurance coverage has expired for sixty-three days or more, your next employer's insurance plan does not have to immediately cover you for any of your pre-existing medical conditions. Consider discussing these issues with your employer's human resources department. Beginning in January 2014, one of the mandates of the Affordable Care Act (ACA) is for insurance companies to cover you for pre-existing medical problems, but time will tell how this turns out.

The good news is that if your company has at least twenty employees and you lose your job, you are allowed to extend your health care benefits under the COBRA law for up to eighteen months. (COBRA stands for Consolidated Omnibus Budget Reconciliation Act.) With COBRA, you can usually continue to receive the group rate, which is often less than purchasing a new individual insurance policy. Nevertheless, continuing your insurance under COBRA can be expensive. But if you or a family member has serious health problems, it is usually advisable to continue your insurance under COBRA because one illness can lead to bankruptcy and accompanying emotional stress. And if you drop your insurance, a new policy with a different insurance company may not cover you for pre-existing medical problems.

Note that there is a thirty-day grace period after employment ends during which you can sign up for COBRA with no interruption in coverage. Pay the premiums on time because some companies will drop your coverage for one late payment.

If your eighteen months of COBRA insurance expires and you are still unemployed, consider buying an individual plan. It may not be too expensive, especially if you are young and healthy and choose a high-deductible plan. You can check with your insurance agent or get quotes from the Internet site www.ehealthinsurance.com.

Also, find out whether you qualify for Medicaid. If you are disabled, look into Social Security's Supplemental Security Income (SSI) and Medicare insurance, even though it often takes considerable time and perseverance.

Some states provide subsidized special high-risk medical insurance pools that insure those with previous health problems and low incomes. Some of these plans have no deductibles or co-payments.

Your options for obtaining medical insurance may improve as major portions of the Affordable Care Act take effect in January 2014.

4

Rights You Have as a Patient

Y ou and I and most Americans rarely take the time to learn the many rights we have as patients. Why? Among other reasons, we assume and trust that the doctor, the hospital, and our other health professionals always act in our best interest. So when we are asked to sign consent forms for diagnostic tests and even for surgery, for example, we may not take the time to read carefully what we are consenting to.

When we are young and healthy, we have a tendency to think we are invulnerable, even immortal. We don't consider our vulnerability and the finiteness of life. We might be reminded of feelings of vulnerability when we watch skydivers or see motorcyclists riding without a helmet. When we are middle aged, we put off or "forget" making a will, filling out legal documents regarding end-of-life decisions, and choosing someone to make health care decisions on our behalf should we become incapacitated. Just as Scarlett O'Hara said in *Gone With the Wind*, "I'll think about that tomorrow."

The following is an example of how our faith in health care professions can influence our decision making.

If you are admitted to a hospital, you are asked to sign reams of paperwork--your agreement to be admitted to the hospital and the consent forms for diagnostic tests, perhaps even for surgery. You may be ill and/or in pain, don't feel clear-headed, are nervous about what's going to happen next, and feel pressure to sign everything quickly so your doctor can get on with things. And you may assume that what you are signing must be in your best interests.

But your rights as a patient entitle you to a clear explanation of the forms you are asked to sign. Take your time to understand them; do not feel rushed. This is a good time to ask for help from your trusted patient advocate and/or a family member who has accompanied you to the hospital. Both of you should ask questions about anything that seems unclear. If time pressures don't permit adequate review, ask the medical staff to summarize the forms. Just as you would want a lawyer to review important legal documents before you sign them, you can request help when you're asked to sign consent forms, especially at a time when you are upset or otherwise preoccupied.

Although it is unpleasant to think about and plan what we want done or not done when facing end-of-life issues, consider taking another approach to these issues that may help you overcome your natural inclination to "think about it tomorrow." You might think about it this way: Dealing with these decisions now helps our family, friends, and physicians know how we want to be treated should we suddenly have to cope with a terminal illness. It also sets a good example for our adult children, who will someday have to confront the realities of life and death. Clearly making our wishes known to those we select (our proxies) to faithfully carry them out lightens the burden on them and conveys our thankfulness for their help.

This chapter provides a brief history of the development of patients' rights and protections, and it summarizes exactly what rights we have and how best to exercise them. It discusses the importance of having a living will, known in many states as a health care advance directive, and it discusses a health care durable power of attorney (also known as a durable power of attorney for health care) and a durable power of attorney for financial decisions. It recommends what to consider when selecting the proxies for these important roles.

This chapter also discusses how to make three important end-of-life decisions: whether or not to initiate Do Not Resuscitate (DNR), Do Not Intubate (DNI) orders, whether or not to have an autopsy, and whether or not to donate your organs or body to benefit science. I share examples from patients and from my personal and family life regarding how we, as patients, make these difficult decisions.

Confidentiality between doctor and patient is one of the oldest and most important rights you have as a patient. It was first advocated by Hippocrates, the Greek philosopher and father of medicine, in about 400 BC. So confidentiality has a long history.

In the United States, many documents have enumerated the rights we all have as patients. In 1973, the American Hospital Association developed the "Patient's Bill of Rights." The Joint Commission on Accreditation of Healthcare Organizations (JCAHO) later developed patient's rights, which hospitals need to honor to maintain their accreditation. In 1997, the Consumer Bill of Rights and Responsibilities was established. In 2003, a major step was taken to protect patients' privacy and confidentiality when Congress passed the Health Insurance Portability and Accountability Act (HIPAA).

These documents ensure and protect your right to:

1. Obtain current, understandable information from your health care professionals regarding your diagnosis, treatment options, progress, prognosis, and estimated medical costs.

2. Have the above explained in a way you can understand if you speak another language, are disabled, or have a hearing loss.

3. Receive respectful, considerate care.

4. Know the roles and identities of all the health professionals involved in your care.

5. Agree or refuse proposed tests and treatments.

6. Agree or refuse to participate in research studies.

7. Review your medical records, have their contents explained, and propose changes if you disagree.

8. Have your medical information be kept confidential except when laws require it be reported (for example, a communicable disease that could endanger the public).

9. Have a living will (health care advance directive) and a durable power of attorney for health care and for financial decisions.

10. Determine what you want done or not done if you become terminally ill.

11. Determine whether or not you want to donate your organs and/or body to benefit science.

In 2003, HIPAA expanded your right to inspect, obtain copies of, and suggest changes to your medical records (after signing a release-of-information form). Your doctor(s) and hospital may ask you to specify what information you want. If your request to make corrections to your record is denied, you can have your request added to your file.

HIPAA also allows you to specify to whom you want your records sent for certain purposes (for example, to have your records shared with your other medical specialists or your new primary care physician). If you think that the confidentiality of your medical records has been violated, you can file an official complaint with your doctor's office, insurance company, and/or hospital. If you are not satisfied with their response, you can also complain to the Health and Human Services Office of

Civil Rights---www.hhs.gov/ocr/civilrights/index.html, or call 1-800-368-1019.

Recent HIPAA rules released in January 2013, known as the "Omnibus Rule," protect your privacy in an ever-expanding digital age. Some of the largest breaches reported to the Department of Health and Human Services (HHS) have involved business associates of providers and insurance companies. These new rules extend current privacy requirements that pertain to health care providers and insurance companies to the business associates of these entities (such as medical equipment manufacturers and computer engineers who install electronic medical records) who have access to your protected health information. The new rules set limits on how information is used and disclosed for marketing and fund-raising purposes.

The Omnibus Rule also strengthens the Health Information Technology for Economic and Clinical Health (HITECH) Breach Notification requirements by clarifying when breaches of health information must be reported. Also, you can ask for a copy of your medical records in electronic form, although as of May 2013 only about half of physician offices were equipped to use electronic medical records. You can also request copies of your written medical records.

Although HIPAA and other patients' rights documents protect your privacy, some information may nevertheless be made available to your insurance company, or be made available in case of a lawsuit or other legal matters. Even in those circumstances, you are usually asked to sign a consent form authorizing release of your records.

A major complaint about HIPAA is that it can act as a double-edged sword. For example, by protecting your records so securely, your new primary care physician (pcp) or the emergency room physician may not have immediate access to crucial information about you, as the following examples illustrate.

I recently interviewed a fifty-year-old woman with a medical problem that was treated by her physician in another city. She signed the consent form allowing her physician to discuss her case with me (her psychiatrist). When I called her physician, he insisted I send or fax the form to him, to comply with HIPAA regulations, before he could discuss the patient. This delayed important changes in her treatment.

For eight years I had been treating a depressed, fatigued woman who was using continuous oxygen. She was referred to a pulmonary specialist in a distant city. The specialist wanted her to sign release-of-information forms and personally gather and send copies of her medical records from her four specialists in Santa Fe. She asked me for a copy of her four-inch-thick chart. Realizing that her pulmonary specialist would not have time to read my records, she signed a consent form permitting me to send a brief summary. It would have been less demanding and time consuming for her if her Santa Fe specialists could have simply called or sent a summarizing e-mail to her consultant.

Because your confidential medical information may be scattered among your various health professionals, what are some ways that it can be made more readily available to your new pcp or to an emergency room physician who knows little about you?

You can make certain that your current pcp and specialists have your written consent to share your medical information with not only your current health professionals but with all health professionals you may see in the future. For example, you can specify---"I give consent to Dr. James Jones to release my medical records to health care professionals I may see from 2013 to 2018." When you see a new physician who wants your former records, he or she will want you to sign a release-of-information form.

It is especially important to sign this consent form before your discharge from the hospital to facilitate timely communication about your hospital stay to your pcp and other health professionals to ensure continuity of care.

Another strategy is to request and personally keep copies in a secure place of all your current medical records and, if relevant, hospital discharge summaries in the event you change doctors, move to another city, or visit an emergency room.

Presently, a Smartphone or other electronic devices can be used to store your medical information (after you have gathered it all) on a special computer chip, so that if you move to a new city or need emergency care, your medical information can be readily accessed. If you choose to use such an electronic device, find out what kind of security is available should you lose the device or computer chip.

The U.S. Department of Health and Human Services has been working for years to create a National Health Information Network (NHIN) to make a person's health records accessible on the Internet. Safeguards need to be in place to protect patient privacy. Once initiated, the NHIN will facilitate better and faster communication between your current and future health providers, reduce health care costs by avoiding unnecessary duplication of expensive tests, and improve treatment outcomes. You will need to keep your computer chip, thumb drive, or Smartphone in a safe place to ensure your privacy.

Living Will, or Health Care Advance Directive

A living will, also known as a health care advance directive, is an important legal document for ensuring the kind of care you want or don't want when facing end-of-life decisions. It is best to make these "advance" decisions when you are well, thinking rationally, and have peace of mind.

Unfortunately, 80 percent of Americans do not have a health care advance directive, and not just because it may seem unnatural to think about what you want your medical team to do or not do should you need to make end-of-life decisions.

You may not have an advance directive for other reasons because (1) your physician may incorrectly assume that you and your attorney have already executed an advance directive; (2) you may not be given the best advice about how to fill out the advance directive forms if your family member, physician, or health care advocate is too busy or distracted to help, or has strong opinions about end-of-life issues; and (3) the simple forms you can download from the Internet may not address the changing status of your complex medical condition.

In addition, we don't always remember to update our advance directive even though our views and wishes may change as we get older and have a different perspective on life. Our advance directive may contain vague instructions. All these potential problems can cause confusion and conflicts among our doctors and family members. As a result, our true wishes may not be followed, leading to prolonged hospitalization, unnecessary aggressive care that may be inconsistent with our true preferences, potential legal arguments between the hospital medical staff and our family, and disputes among our family members who may be pressured by hospital staff to make decisions on our behalf.

An advance directive comes into effect only when it is determined by our physician (sometimes with the help of a medical consultant) that we no longer have the mental capacity to make end-of-life decisions. If our mental capacity for making these decisions is restored and this is substantiated by our physician, then our most current wishes will be respected.

If you want to change your advance directive, you will need to fill out a new directive, and give copies to your doctor, attorney, health care proxy, patient advocate, and selected family members. Be sure to tear up all copies of your previous directive. Advance directives usually require one or two witnesses to attest that you are personally known to them and are of sound mind when you sign the document.

You have a number of options when you review an advance directive. For example, you can state that you voluntarily and willfully want (or do not want) your moment of death to be artificially postponed if your physician and medical staff thinks that your illness is terminal. You can request withholding death-delaying procedures, such as being intubated, connected to a respirator, or being resuscitated, which would only prolong the dying process. Furthermore, you can state that you be permitted to die naturally with only administration of pain and other medication and nutrition deemed necessary by your physician to provide you with comfort care.

On the other hand, should you want all efforts exercised by your medical team to keep you alive--including, if needed, the use of a respirator and being resuscitated--you can indicate these wishes in your advance directive. If you do not have an advance directive and do not fill one out before or during hospitalization or a stay in a nursing home indicating that you do not want death-delaying procedures performed, then the hospital or nursing home staff will most likely attempt to resuscitate you, often causing you great discomfort, little likelihood of regaining a reasonable quality of life, and tremendous expense.

The following case illustrates these points. A ninety-year-old woman who had suffered a stroke four years earlier, causing an inability to express herself, was admitted to the hospital with a fractured hip, advanced cancer, and an inability to eat. Because she could not speak, her hospitalist misdiagnosed her as "demented." Her family insisted on having a feeding tube inserted. A few days later the advance directive that she had completed five years earlier (before her stroke) was found. It stated: "I do not want to be fed artificially if two physicians certify that I have an incurable illness and determine that death is imminent and life-sustaining procedures would only artificially prolong the dying process." A geriatric consultant was able to use hand signs to communicate with her and found she was not demented but demonstrated full capacity to make her own medical decisions. She was adamant about not wanting a feeding tube. Her wishes were honored, and her family agreed.

Because she had an advance directive and was currently capable of making an informed decision, her wishes were respected.

Appendix I has a sample of a Health Care Advance Directive and a form for appointing a health care power of attorney that is used in the state of New Mexico. Appendix II has a sample of a Physician Orders for Life-Sustaining Treatment (POLST) form used in California that is signed by you or a legally recognized decision maker, such as your health care proxy, and your physician, which indicates what you want done or not done regarding end of life decisions. Fill out similar forms that are specific for the state where you live. Update your POLST and Health Care Advance Directive periodically to ensure consistency and to reflect your current wishes.

It's advisable to make a copy of the POLST or similar forms for your state and keep it in your wallet in case of an emergency. Because many patients do not have a lawyer and haven't executed an advance directive, the POLST or similar form is a perfect option. You can type "POLST" into your Internet browser to obtain more information about the form used in your state.

If you presently don't have an advance directive or have one that needs updating, meet with your pcp, your attorney, or an administrator at your nearby hospital to complete a comprehensive advance directive that clearly states your wishes.

If you have never filled out an advance directive and are admitted to a hospital or nursing home, your doctor or staff member will give you forms similar to the POLST to specify whether or not you want life-sustaining measures instituted. These forms are routinely given to all patients who do not have an advance directive, so don't perceive it as preparation for a dire outcome.

Because state laws differ, should you move to another state, complete a new advance directive that conforms to that state's requirements with the assistance of an attorney, doctor, or hospital administrator. When I moved from Illinois to New

Mexico, I met with my new attorney, who advised me to fill out a new advance directive that conformed to New Mexico law, to send copies to all who needed to know my wishes, and to destroy my previous directive.

Health Care Durable Power of Attorney

Also known as a durable power of attorney for health care, this document appoints a person and an alternate health care proxy of your choosing to make important medical decisions on your behalf if you become incapacitated and/or no longer have the mental capacity to make these decisions. It's important to designate someone you trust and who knows you well. The person you select should fully understand and have a copy of your advance directive and also clearly understand what you want and don't want done by your medical team if your clinical condition changes. Situations often arise during your treatment that are not fully covered in your advance directive, so your health care proxy should understand what you would want or not want done and communicate your wishes to your medical team. Make sure that all your health care professionals, your patient advocate, attorney, and selected family members have a copy of your durable power of attorney. Bring a copy of your advance directive and durable power of attorney with you if you require hospitalization.

Deciding Who to Designate

Designating a health care proxy helps to avoid arguments about health care decisions among your family members and friends. Even though your spouse is legally considered your next of kin and is often chosen as your proxy for health care decisions, you can select someone else. You want someone who is readily accessible, has ample time to stay informed about your changing medical status, stays calm and rational under stress, and is knowledgeable about your finances and insurance coverage should a decision need to be made about what you can afford if post-hospital rehabilitation or nursing home care is needed. Your proxy should have good communication skills to discuss your condition with your physician and other health professionals (such as a social worker) and be tactful in discussing your condition and treatment options with family members (some of whom may have opposing views).

Years ago I had designated my adult daughter as my health care proxy, but she became involved with legal difficulties of another family member and also had a busy career. Meanwhile, my son had graduated from medical school. After discussing with him my strong feelings about not wanting heroic measures carried out should I become terminally ill, I decided to designate him as my principal proxy with my daughter as alternate. It's advisable to appoint a secondary proxy should your first proxy's circumstances change, such as becoming geographically inaccessible or ill. I could see the disappointment on my daughter's face when I explained my decision, pointing out that this would relieve her of yet another responsibility. She understood and was not resentful.

If you do not have a relative or friend to serve as your proxy, you can ask your attorney, your hospital's administrator, or a social worker for candidates to interview. Learn about the potential proxy's experience, fees, and arrangements for payment. After selecting your proxy, explain thoroughly your wishes regarding future health care decisions, your financial and insurance information (whether or not you have home care and/or nursing home insurance), and which friends and family members you would want notified were you to become ill.

Your health care proxy (along with your alternate proxy) needs to be officially noted in the power of attorney documents. Give a copy of the form that designates your health care proxy and a copy of your advance directive, to your physician, patient advocate, and selected family members so everyone is aware of his or her role and responsibilities.

Your Responsibilities as Health Care Proxy

One assumes the role of health care proxy only if your relative or friend becomes seriously ill and lacks the capacity to make health care decisions. Your role can be a formidable one. Should your friend or relative be hospitalized, you need to establish good rapport with the attending physician and other health professionals (especially the social worker) so you have up-to-date knowledge to share with relatives and friends. Let hospital staff and family members know about your role, and have a copy of the form that designates you as health care proxy, and a copy of the health care directive. Should the physician determine that your friend or relative is incapacitated, be prepared to participate in decisions about his or her hospital and post-hospital care.

Being active in your role as health care proxy is appreciated by the doctors and other health professionals because they can concentrate their efforts on helping your relative recover and be relieved of some of the burden of answering questions from many family members and friends. As proxy, you can be under considerable strain because you are dealing with your own grief and sadness witnessing your relative's decline while tending to similar emotional reactions of family and friends and simultaneously discussing medical and other decisions with the doctors, social worker, and other professionals. Keep in mind that you are making decisions reflecting your relative's wishes and not your own. This may assuage some psychological anguish and guilt if you are expressing your terminally ill relative's desire to die in peace rather than be kept alive with heroic measures.

Durable Power of Attorney for Financial Decisions

Similar to designating someone to make health care decisions should you become incapacitated, select someone (and an alternate) to make financial decisions on your behalf should you become unable to make such decisions yourself. Your attorney, hospital administrator, and social worker or the Internet can provide state-specific documents for you to fill out that designate who you select as your financial proxy and an alternate.

Should you become incapacitated, your financial proxy needs to know all about your estate and finances or how to obtain this information (such as from your attorney, accountant, financial advisor, and/or your secure fireproof file cabinet). I selected my oldest son, who possesses all this information and because he's knowledgeable about financial planning and has met my attorney and accountant. His brother (the doctor) is proxy for medical decisions. They understand what roles they will both assume were that to become necessary.

My attorney and I have agreed that were I to become incapacitated, she would arrange a meeting (in person or by conference call) with my three adult children and my accountant to decide on current and future health care and financial decisions that would need to be made on my behalf. They would communicate when unpredictable situations arose.

Every few years I write a letter to my attorney and three adult children with a complete update of any major changes in my financial situation and health care providers (such as a change to a new pcp). My son who is my financial proxy has authority to sign checks on my behalf, take care of current bills, has access to my safety deposit box, a key to my home, and has the authority to take over other financial responsibilities.

You may want to consider some of the above planning strategies that are most pertinent to you and your family.

Do Not Resuscitate (DNR), Do Not Intubate (DNI)

When you are well and thinking rationally is the best time to fill out legal forms (with help of your pcp or patient advocate) regarding your health care directive. You can indicate whether or not you want lifesaving measures, such as being intubated and resuscitated if your heart or breathing fails. If you don't have a health care directive and are hospitalized or admitted to a nursing home and are capable of making health care decisions, you can fill out forms similar to the POLST. If your condition is terminal and you don't want to be resuscitated, you should sign forms expressing these wishes (DNR/DNI). Otherwise, the medical team will probably do everything they can to resuscitate you, which would probably only prolong your suffering and increase expenses. If your condition improves and you have the mental capacity to decide that you now want lifesaving measures to be instituted, you can rescind the DNR/DNI request.

Donation of Organs and Issue of an Autopsy

If you were to die suddenly, do you want your viable organs to be donated to a needy recipient? Do you want to have an autopsy? Understandably, many people, for religious and personal reasons, feel uncomfortable subjecting their bodies for these purposes.

The potential benefit of subjecting your body to an autopsy is to provide your children with more information about the risks of developing an inheritable disease (should you be found to have one), and to be more knowledgeable about your health conditions and any precautions they can take to avoid such illnesses. An autopsy can also educate your medical team about possible diagnostic or treatment errors that can save future lives and advance medical knowledge.

In some states, you can indicate on your driver's license whether or not you want to donate organs in case you were to die in an auto accident. Whatever your wishes, you need to sign the appropriate documents. You can discuss these issues with your attorney or a social worker at your nearby hospital.

PART III

5

Assuming More Responsibility for Your Health Care

T his chapter suggests ways for overcoming barriers to a healthier lifestyle and ways of assuming more responsibility for your and your family's health care. There are preventive measures that you and your family can implement right now for getting and staying healthy throughout all stages of life, beginning in childhood and continuing through the senior years.

Remember when your doctor could spend as much time with you as necessary? He or she felt obvious pride, responsibility, and autonomy in caring for you and other family members.

The now almost obsolete concept of a "house call" was commonplace when I was growing up. When we were too sick to go to the doctor's office, our family's physician came to the house. In those days, doctors were revered and highly respected by their patients.

While practicing medicine and psychiatry for twenty-three years in Chicago, I had an excellent old-fashioned physician who spent an hour with me carrying out my yearly medical checkup, including a half-hour physical examination, which included listening to my heart and chest, palpating my abdomen, and examining my prostate. He personally called me with the results of the tests; his assistant always scheduled a follow-up appointment.

What happened to change the bedside manner of the family physician? Big business happened. It became the intermediary between you -- the patient -- and your doctor. Medical insurance and managed care are two examples of big business intruding into the doctor-patient relationship.

Today, in America's fragmented health care system, doctors are pressured to see more patients for shorter periods of time. Although they continue to feel morally bound to be the best physicians they were trained to be, they find themselves spending 20 percent or more of their valuable time doing administrative work, such as telephoning for insurance authorizations and filling out endless paperwork. Low reimbursements from insurance companies and government programs such as Medicaid and Medicare have not kept up with the increased costs of running a medical practice. Some doctors find themselves practicing defensive medicine to avoid a malpractice suit.

These pressures account for the dissatisfaction and demoralization of physicians and their staff—feelings that are sometimes expressed by impatience and harried behavior with patients. Busy, pressured physicians don't find the time to communicate with their patients' other physicians and health professionals, yet these are important tasks to ensure coordinated care. These frustrations have led many physicians to cease being Medicare, Medicaid, and managed care providers.

Consequently, you and I need to be even more conscientious, proactive, and responsible for our medical and mental health care. To ensure that you and I are getting the best care possible, consider these three suggestions. (1) Recognize the fragmentation and deficiencies of our current health care system. (2) Be more knowledgeable and inquisitive about your diagnosis and treatment by making use of reliable Internet sites and other educational resources. (3) Ask questions of your health care team, and repeat them until you feel confident that you understand the answers.

The "Not Me" Phenomenon

What prevents us from taking charge of our health care? Believe it or not, one of the biggest factors is our own psychological barriers—the emotional and psychological roadblocks we all share.

What are some of these psychological barriers? First, it is scary and anxiety producing to think we are vulnerable to a minor illness, not to mention a serious one. When we are young and healthy, it is normal and natural to believe in one's invincibility and invulnerability. We don't even think about our mortality, much less feel the need to come to grips with it. Unless challenged by personal or family illness or other serious life events, we usually continue to think this way as we get older.

Second, we all share to some degree common psychological defense mechanisms such as denial, suppression, and/or rationalization. All these reinforce the belief that we are not vulnerable to the slings and arrows of misfortune, such as medical illness. Denial helps us avoid the awareness of some painful aspect of reality--such as symptoms of a medical illness--by negating sensory data (for example, discomfort from a persistent cough). Using suppression, we consciously or semiconsciously postpone attention to a conscious concern or conflict (for example, the persistent cough). We acknowledge the discomfort, but we minimize it. Using rationalization, we offer explanations to justify beliefs or behavior (for example, my cough will go away if I ignore it). We often just procrastinate. These normal (and--if used excessively--detrimental) defenses reinforce the "not me" phenomenon. And they get in the way of a proactive approach to our health care. We pay a price by using these natural defense mechanisms excessively because they interfere with early recognition of symptoms and prevent us from seeking early medical intervention.

Third, it is more pleasant to plan our vacation, retirement, or our child's upcoming graduation than to plan for the possibility of a serious illness.

What follows is another example of how these defense mechanisms can interfere with early intervention . A thirty-four-year-old woman notices a swelling in her breast but tells herself it's nothing and doesn't give it a second thought (denial). Months later the swelling has increased, but she consciously decides not to give it much attention (suppression). The swelling increases further, but she ascribes it to having bumped into something, which explains the initial swelling (rationalization), so she puts off seeing her doctor (procrastination).

How to Overcome Psychological Barriers

Here are a few suggestions for overcoming these psychological barriers. It's important to start the process now because psychological barriers interfere with being prepared if you or family members are stricken with a medical problem.

The first step is to seriously think about your personal psychological makeup and recognize the normal tendency to deny, suppress, "keep out of mind," and use other protective psychological mechanisms to avoid recognizing early symptoms of a medical or psychological problem.

Second, Just Do It. Start in the same way you would plan a vacation or save for retirement. Compile a comprehensive profile of health care information that includes all your significant past and current medical problems and all the medications you are taking. Your health care profile is essential when you visit your physician, go to an emergency room or urgent care center, or are admitted to a hospital. Enlist the help of a family member or a friend, and promise to return the favor. The process is tedious and time consuming, but one day it may save your life. And it will set a good example for your children, other family members, and friends. The Affordable Care Act (ACA) won't solve all the problems of our fragmented health care system, so take more responsibility for your own health care now.

Third, enlist the services of a health care coach or trainer, or join an exercise group at your local gym. They can help you develop a personalized exercise program, diet, and other ways of adopting a healthier lifestyle. When you do your part, you give the health care system, imperfect as it is, the best chance to work for you.

Preparing for Your Initial Visit: Your Health Care Profile

The first step in preparing your health care profile is to assemble a comprehensive health history so this important information can be shared, in a team-like fashion, with your doctor, other health professionals, and the hospital staff (if you are admitted to a hospital). Whether preparing for a routine or an urgent visit to your physician, have this information handy. It should include a detailed list of your current symptoms-- when they started, how long they lasted, where the pain and/or other symptoms are located, whether the symptoms are mild, moderate, or severe, what makes the symptoms worse or better, and what medications have been tried--and their effectiveness.

Your health care profile should also include a list of questions to ask your doctor. Office visits have become briefer in recent years, and normal tension and anxiety may cause you to forget important details. Whenever possible, bring a family member or your health care advocate to your doctor's appointment. Your advocate may ask questions that you've forgotten and be another set of ears to ensure that you adhere to the treatment plan. Request a follow-up appointment to discuss the results of any tests and your response to treatment.

Aids to Compiling Your Health Care Profile

By now you are probably asking yourself how you can possibly convey all this information to your doctor, especially given the brevity of most doctor visits. Fortunately, many doctors' offices will send you questionnaires to fill out prior to your initial appointment, which will allow you more time for discussion during the actual appointment. When you arrange your first appointment, ask the doctor's office to send you these forms.

Also, there are Internet sites where you can store all your information (and that of other family members) online so your doctor, or anyone you give permission to, can access this information from any location. Useful Internet sites include the Joint Commission Resources own web site (www.jcrinc.com) and www.webmd.com/health-manager. Some sites charge a nominal fee. Smartphones and other electronic devices can store all your medical information on a computer chip, but learn what security measures are available to protect your privacy.

Whether you decide to organize your health care information on your own, on the Internet, on electronic devices, or on forms supplied by your doctor, include as much of the following information as possible:

1. Significant past illnesses and your response to treatment.

2. Allergies to medications, foods, and other allergens such as plants.

3. Illnesses that your parents, siblings, grandparents, and great-grandparents had. (You can construct a family tree to hold this information.) Some illnesses (such as diabetes, heart disease, schizophrenia, mood disorders, or cancer) may make you genetically predisposed to the same illnesses. If a family member was never given a diagnosis, ask another family member what the symptoms

were (for example, depressed mood or impaired memory). When compiling this family history, don't be shy about asking for information from other family members, especially someone who's proud of being the family historian.

If several close family members had illnesses that are genetically transmissible (such as diabetes), ask your doctor how likely you are to inherit the condition, and what you can do to prevent it (for example, diet, exercise, weight control).

4. Record the habits of family members and friends with whom you had close contact over considerable time. Their habits (smoking, high-cholesterol diets, exposure to toxins such as lead or uranium) can potentially have a detrimental effect on you.

One final suggestion: Keep in your wallet or purse at all times a brief summary of all this important information, especially your current medications and allergies. Include several emergency contact persons (reliable relatives, your advocate) in case you find yourself in an emergency room or a hospital. This information will then be readily available to those responsible for your care.

Getting and Staying Healthy Throughout All Stages of Life

Perhaps the surest way to avoid dealing with an imperfect health care system is to adopt a healthy lifestyle. We all know that following a healthy lifestyle will reduce your risk for acute and chronic diseases, help you be more resilient should you become ill, and increase your longevity.

Why do so few people follow a healthy lifestyle? Americans have one of the highest rates of obesity in the world. Many of us do not eat nutritional foods, exercise regularly, sleep at least six to seven hours a night, take nutritional supplements (vitamins and minerals), or have sufficient meaning and purpose in life. A healthy lifestyle means fewer doctor visits, medications, and hospitalizations—all of which are fraught with risks.

The following are some of many reasons why Americans don't practice scientifically proven ways of staying healthy and living longer. Think seriously about which of the following obstacles stand in your way. It is never too late to change.

1. Lack of Role Models

If you grew up in a family that didn't practice a healthy lifestyle, you probably didn't eat healthy food or exercise because we tend to be influenced by those closest to us. During adolescence, peer pressure makes us conform to our group's lifestyle. If these role models don't practice principles of healthy living, where will we learn them?

2. Fast-Paced American Lifestyle and Stressful Economic Times

The pressure on the middle and lower class to sustain a living during difficult economic times leads to shortened mealtimes and the choice of inexpensive, non-nutritional fast food that is high in calories, salt, fat, and sugar--a recipe leading to obesity and all its complications.

3. The "Not Me" Phenomenon

We all have a tendency to want instant gratification, including denial of the long-term health consequences of an unhealthy lifestyle. We are more apt to order chocolate cake rather than fruit on a restaurant's dessert menu because of the immediate gratification after a strenuous day at work. We all find ways of rationalizing our less than healthy choices.

4. Medical and Mental Health Problems

Obesity or depression may deter you from beginning an exercise program at a gym because of self-consciousness and apathy. Exercise is known to combat depression by stimulating the brain's production of endorphins and mood-enhancing neurotransmitters. Depression has been shown to interfere with cooperating with medical treatment, such as reliably attending follow-up visits with your physician.

Many aspects of the ACA are designed to help us avoid the risks of diabetes, hypertension, heart disease, stroke, and other debilitating and costly illnesses. Major portions of the ACA that will come into effect in 2014 emphasize preventative health care programs and healthier ways of living to encourage us to get and stay healthy throughout all stages of our lives.

6

Finding a Qualified Primary Care Physician, Psychiatrist, and Other Medical Specialist

B renda worked in a factory in a medium-size midwestern city. Her employer contracted with a new health insurance company to reduce costs. Brenda had an excellent relationship over the past eighteen years with her internist, who was not a provider with her company's new insurer. Brenda learned that there were a limited number of physicians in her community who were providers with the new insurer and even fewer who were accepting new patients.

She asked the human resources department of her company for a list of primary care physicians (pcp's) with contracts with the new insurer. She called these physicians, only to learn that some had retired. Some were no longer taking new patients, and those who were did not have openings for several months. She felt frustrated and was at a loss as to what to do.

Perhaps you or your family members have had similar problems finding a new physician. This chapter offers useful strategies for finding a pcp or a specialist such as a psychiatrist despite obstacles that may stand in your way. These strategies can be applied to finding other medical specialists.

It is crucial to find a physician you can depend upon and trust and with whom you can form a long-lasting relationship. Unfortunately, there is a shortage of physicians in the United

States, an insufficient number graduating from medical and osteopathic schools, and a longtime shortage of those practicing in rural areas. Not enough medical school graduates are going into primary care fields of medicine, such as family practice, internal medicine, general practice, and pediatrics. The current shortage of pcp's will become more acute as increasing numbers of uninsured Americans, under the Affordable Care Act (ACA) in January 2014, become eligible for Medicaid and insurance via exchanges, in addition to the rapidly expanding baby boomer generation eligible for Medicare.

Unfortunately, an increasing number of pcp's are limiting the number of new Medicare and Medicaid patients they admit into their practice, and many are no longer providers for these government programs. Yet most insurance plans, especially managed care companies, require patients to have a pcp who serves the important role of coordinating a patient's overall care and making referrals to specialists. Your pcp is responsible for having a comprehensive knowledge of not only your medical problems and history but also your psychological and social situation – somewhat like the old-fashioned country doctor.

You want to feel that your pcp is genuinely interested in you, is reliable and available, and knows the best experts if referral to a specialist becomes necessary. The physician you select, and the office staff, need good organizational skills so your medical care is integrated with care provided by your other physicians and health care providers.

In deciding who you want as your pcp, consider inquiring (from the physician or the physician's nurse assistant) the extent of the physician's training and experience treating the problems you have. You also want to know who provides coverage when the physician is unavailable, and who will take care of you should hospitalization ever become necessary.

Finding the Physician Who Is Right for You

Good sources for selecting a pcp are friends and relatives, especially those who work in the health care field who are knowledgeable about the physician's qualifications. You can also call your insurance or managed care company for a list of pcp's near you. Sometimes these lists are outdated, or don't specify whether the physician is accepting new patients, and don't provide the physician's background and experience. To find "Dr. Right," you need to be persistent, patient, and prepared to make numerous telephone calls.

Another good source is the Internet. If you don't have a computer at home, you can use one at any public library. The American Medical Association's web site, www.ama-assn.org, lets you search for doctors by medical specialty or name. It also has a "group practice locator" site that lets you search for group practices by state.

Another Internet site, sponsored by the American Association of Family Physicians (AAFP), lets you search for family practice physicians by zip code. Another source is Medline Plus (www.medlineplus.gov), sponsored by the National Institutes of Health (NIH) and the U.S. National Library of Medicine, which has resources for finding hospitals, doctors, and dentists.

There are advantages to selecting physicians who are Board certified because they have passed rigorous examinations in their specialty, which validates their knowledge and skill. There are, however, highly qualified physicians who, for various reasons, may have opted not to take the exam required for Board certification. A physician listed as Board eligible has not yet taken the examination or has failed it. To find out whether the doctor you are considering is Board certified, check www.abms.org, or call the American Board of Medical Specialists at 866-275-2267. If you have one or two physicians as possible candidates, you can use an Internet browser such as google.com and enter the physicians' names to obtain information about their training, experience, and publishing history.

If you are determined to enlist the services of a particular physician, here are strategies to achieve your objective. If the office manager tells you that the doctor is not accepting new patients, ask if you could be placed on a waiting list or if you could be seen if a scheduled patient cancels. If relatives or friends are his or her patients, mention their name. Use your interpersonal skills to get to know the office manager. Call a few days later to see if a scheduled patient canceled and an opening has become available.

Don't be shy about making important inquires about the doctor you are considering. For example, if you're told that this doctor is the managing physician of a large group practice and sees patients infrequently, you may want to use another doctor in the group.

If the physician you want is not available even after trying these strategies, ask the office manager to recommend other physicians.

Here are additional questions to consider asking your prospective physician's office staff.

1. Do other physicians and their families use the doctor for their care?

2. How old is the doctor? Is he or she nearing retirement or planning to move to a new locale? There are advantages to seeing someone younger than yourself, to reduce the chances of your outliving him or her. And younger physicians may be more knowledgeable about newer treatments.

3. Does the doctor treat a lot of patients with medical illnesses similar to yours?

The major take-home message here is this: If you find a pcp you value, do what you can to continue under that physician's care.

An increasing number of physicians have not only ceased being providers for (or opted out of) Medicare and Medicaid but have elected, for various reasons, not to be a provider with any insurance company. These physicians are then referred to as "out-of-network" or non-participating doctors. You pay them directly for their services. Before making an appointment, ask your insurance company whether or not and to what extent you would be entitled to partial reimbursement from your insurance company if you submit a detailed bill marked "paid" from your out-of-network (or non-participating) physician. The amount you may be reimbursed varies widely, so it's helpful to know in advance. You can also ask your insurance company if they would authorize you to see the out-of-network physician as a single-case exemption. Out-of-network doctors are often reluctant to take on a single-case exemption because of the tremendous amount of paperwork involved.

If you have Medicare and a secondary insurance but the physician is not a Medicare provider, neither you nor the physician can send a bill to Medicare. But some secondary insurance companies may provide some reimbursement if your physician's office provides you with a detailed paid bill and you submit it to your secondary insurer. Find out the details from your secondary insurer beforehand so there are no surprises. Consider asking your secondary insurance company to put its policy in writing to minimize later misunderstandings when you submit the physician's paid bill.

Some physicians, especially in large metropolitan cities, are not providers with any insurance company. Sometimes referred to as having "boutique practices," doctors are paid a monthly or yearly fee in exchange for being readily available for appointments and telephone consultations. There is usually a separate charge for office visits. There are various agreements regarding services provided and the fees for them.

Finding a Specialist

You may want to consider seeing a specialist if you are not recovering as quickly as expected from your illness, not feeling comfortable with your pcp, or you or a family member intuitively feels that it's time to get a second opinion (discussed in more detail in Chapter 12).

One strategy is to have a frank discussion with your pcp about seeing a specialist. Your pcp knows and works closely with a number of specialists. With your written permission, the pcp sends copies of your records and/or calls the specialist to discuss your case. The specialist's recommendations are communicated to your pcp, who integrates the recommendations into your overall treatment plan.

The role of the pcp is especially important in caring for fragile, elderly patients who often take multiple medications and visit several specialists. All health professionals need to know who is "captain of the ship" and who is responsible for which aspects of the elderly patient's treatment, such as who is responsible for adjusting which medications. Otherwise, treatment becomes fragmented and fraught with errors rather than being integrated and coordinated.

If you choose to consult a specialist on your own, you can get recommendations from friends or relatives in the health care field or use the Internet to find a Board-certified specialist. You, your pcp, and the specialist can decide if it's possible to continue under the specialist's care, continue under the care of your pcp, or utilize the services of both. It's important that all those involved are clear about what role and responsibility each physician will assume.

The following strategies for finding a psychiatrist or other mental health professional are also relevant for finding other specialists.

Finding a Psychiatrist, Mental Health Professional, or Other Medical Specialist

Making an appointment with a psychiatrist or other mental health professional, such as a psychotherapist or a family counselor, can be a challenging, frustrating experience, as illustrated by the following patient.

Julie, an attractive twenty-two-year-old married nurse living in New York City, became very depressed after the birth of her first child. Her pcp put her on an antidepressant and told her to call her insurance company to find a psychiatrist.

The first few she called were not taking new patients; the next four no longer were providers with her insurance company and didn't know psychiatrists who were providers. She and her husband became increasingly frustrated and considered abandoning the search. Finally, she asked her hospital co-workers for a recommendation. A close friend recommended Dr. Clark, who had an excellent reputation but rarely had openings for new patients.

When Dr. Clark explained that he had no available appointments for several months, Julie became assertive and asked if she could call again in a few days to see if he had a cancellation. She was pleased to be able to see him a week later, felt comforted by his gentle, empathic manner, and was on the road to recovery within a few sessions.

Some psychiatrists have special training and experience in treating children, couples, families, or elderly patients and particular types of problems such as depression, anxiety, or substance abuse. In general, psychiatrists tend to treat patients with major psychiatric problems; many such patients require a combination of psychotherapy and medication.

If you are looking for a Board-certified psychiatrist, you can contact the American Board of Medical Specialties or call the district branch of the American Psychiatric Association (APA) near where you live. To find the district branch, call the APA at 1-888-35-psych or go to www.psych.org.

If you have an elderly family member suffering from a psychiatric problem, you can call the American Association for Geriatric Psychiatry to find a geriatric psychiatry specialist (301-654-7850) or go to www.AAGPonline.org.

You can also use the Yellow Pages of your local telephone directory under the heading "Physicians," then look for "Specialists," and then the list of psychiatrists. You can call your insurance company for the names of psychiatrists who are providers with your insurance company. Another alternative is using an Internet browser. Type in the name of the prospective specialist to obtain information about him or her. You can also get a physician's rating from patients who have seen a particular specialist by going to a peer-reviewed web site such as yelp.com or healthgrades.com.

Another way to find a psychiatrist or mental health professional is by calling the psychiatry department of a nearby university medical center. If they have a psychiatric residency training program, there are doctors in training you can see who are supervised by experienced psychiatrists. These psychiatric outpatient clinics accept insurance, and fees are usually on a sliding scale commensurate with your financial situation. Additional resources are state- or county-supported community mental health clinics and Veterans Administration (VA) hospitals and clinics (for veterans who meet certain criteria).

If you live in a small rural community, you are primarily dependent on your pcp for almost all your health care, but your doctor may have access to consultation with a psychiatrist or other specialist in a nearby city. Some rural areas have tele-psychiatry programs, where a patient can be interviewed and treatment can be planned via audiovisual equipment connected from the rural physician's office to a psychiatrist's office or the psychiatry department at a university medical center.

Your pcp is usually capable of treating simple depression and anxiety disorders and will refer those with more serious problems to a psychiatrist. For less serious psychological problems, a state-licensed therapist with a background in psychology, social work, or psychiatric nursing is capable of providing psychotherapy, but the majority of psychotherapists are not licensed to prescribe medication.

In group practices of psychiatrists working in collaboration with psychotherapists, therapy is often provided by the latter, and medication along with some psychotherapy by the former. Patients are asked to sign a consent form permitting the psychiatrist, psychotherapist, and pcp to communicate with one another. If your physician or psychiatrist is referring you to a psychotherapist, sign these consent forms so clinical records arrive or telephone discussions can take place even before your first meeting with the psychotherapist. Communication between psychiatrist and psychotherapist is very important in facilitating a coordinated treatment plan.

Sometimes the psychiatrist and psychotherapist don't know each other, and there is a risk that, for various reasons, the psychiatrist and the psychotherapist may work at cross purposes. So encourage communication between your two health professionals.

Your Initial Call to a Psychiatrist or Other Mental Health Professional

When making the initial call to a prospective psychiatrist, psychotherapist, and other mental health professional, find out if he or she is accepting new patients and is a provider with your insurance company. Briefly explain your main problem.

If you call a psychiatrist who does not have office staff, he or she may ask you to contact your insurance company to find out if you have a yearly deductible and what portion of it you have met and what your co-payment is for a typical forty-five- to fifty-minute session. Understanding your insurance coverage and responsibility before treatment begins avoids later misunderstandings.

The most important take-home message is to decide that you are going to do everything in your power to get the help you need and deserve. Don't entertain old-fashioned stereotypical beliefs that it is shameful, a sign of weakness, or an indication of "craziness" to ask for help from a psychiatrist or a psychotherapist.

More than half of all psychiatric patients don't complete the first few sessions in most community mental health clinics because of these barriers to engaging with a psychiatrist or psychotherapist: discomfort and shame about revealing personal aspects of yourself, cultural biases, ambivalent feelings toward mental health professionals, and transportation and financial limitations. One of the most important determinates of getting well is your willingness to make a commitment to treatment. Studies have shown that patients most likely to benefit from treatment are those who regularly attend their appointments.

The Differences Between a Psychiatrist and a Psychotherapist

A psychiatrist is a physician who, after completing four years of medical school, trains for about four additional years at a psychiatric residency training program. The curriculum includes biological, psychological, sociological, and cultural bases for various psychiatric disorders, the theories and practice of different psychotherapies (insight-oriented, supportive, cognitive-behavioral, interpersonal, family, and others), and the judicious use of psychiatric medications. Because he or she has a medical background, the psychiatrist is knowledgeable about how a medical illness can present as a psychiatric disorder and contribute to psychiatric symptoms. And because the psychiatrist has specialized training in the use and side effects of psychiatric medications, he or she can prescribe these medications, usually in combination with psychotherapy, to treat various psychiatric illnesses (such as mood and anxiety disorders, schizophrenia, behavioral problems of dementia, and addiction).

Many, but not all, psychiatrists take a special examination under the auspices of the American Board of Psychiatry and Neurology to become Board certified in general psychiatry. Some psychiatrists, following successful completion of a four-year residency, elect to train for an additional year or more to become proficient in a subspecialty area, such as child, adolescent, family, or geriatric psychiatry, addiction or forensic psychiatry, and other specialties. Most specialists take an additional examination to become Board certified in that subspecialty. Board-certified psychiatrists with a subspecialty, and other subspecialty physicians, are expected to become recertified in that subspecialty by passing an examination every ten years or so in order to maintain their Board-certified status.

A psychotherapist may have a background in psychology, sociology, nursing, education, or other fields and special training in the theories and practice of various psychotherapies (somewhat like the training of psychiatrists), but they have no medical training. To practice psychotherapy, therapists need to be licensed in the state where they practice.

In contrast to psychiatrists, psychologists are not licensed to prescribe psychiatric medication except in several states (such as New Mexico and Alaska) where psychologists undergo special training and need to pass an examination. In some states, clinical nurse specialists and physician assistants can prescribe psychiatric medication, usually under the supervision of a physician.

7

Preparing to See a Psychiatrist, Psychotherapist, or Other Mental Health Professional

T his chapter focuses on and helps you prepare for your first appointment with a psychiatrist, but it is also relevant to seeing a psychotherapist or other mental health professional. And if you are reluctant to acknowledge a problem and have delayed seeking help, it may also help you determine the causes for your inaction.

Try to become aware of why you may have avoided seeking help in the past. For example, people who are very depressed often feel hopeless and make the false assumption that nothing, including seeing a psychiatrist, will help. Concern about disapproval from family and neighbors may add to one's reluctance. Another impediment may be cultural factors, such as the belief that only "crazy" people or those who are "loco" need to see a psychiatrist.

Even before you call for a doctor's appointment, think about the major reasons you are seeking help. What are the stressful events that led to your emotional upheaval? What are your current symptoms? Asking yourself why you are depressed or anxious helps to identify the current contributing stressors.

Try to recall past episodes of emotional stress that caused similar symptoms and how you coped with and overcame adversity. These memories will remind you of past successful coping strategies and provide some relief and reassurance that can help with your current problems. For example, did working harder at your occupation or talking with a trusted confidant help you during a previous crisis? If you were in therapy in the past, identifying what helped or didn't help will be useful information for the psychiatrist.

Recalling characteristics of a previous helpful psychiatrist will aid in deciding whether or not you can work with the new psychiatrist. There are advantages to returning to the psychiatrist who helped you before because he or she knows your history and past treatment. It is like getting together with a trusted friend with whom you can air your concerns and who once again can be comforting, empathic, and insightful. Do not allow feelings of shame or embarrassment about having a relapse or disappointing your psychiatrist interfere with a return visit.

Selecting a psychiatrist is like choosing your primary care physician (pcp). One needs to feel trust and feel understood in order to build a working alliance. If the psychiatrist reminds you of a conflictual relationship you have had with a significant person from your past, such as a parent or a sibling, discuss this openly to determine whether or not you can work together. And don't be shy about asking about the psychiatrist's training and experience in helping patients with similar problems.

As with your first visit to your pcp, bring a list of all medical and psychiatric medications you are taking, including over-the-counter or herbal medications, because side effects may be contributing to your current symptoms. Your psychiatrist will want to know what psychiatric medications are helping you presently or helped in the past as well as medications that helped other family members because genetic factors can influence how effective the same medication may be for you. Two or even three sessions may be required before the psychiatrist has the necessary information to explain your diagnosis and treatment options.

Have a frank discussion about the treatment agreement. Discuss fees, the psychiatrist's availability between appointments, your responsibility for missed appointments, who covers while he or she is away, and whom to call in an emergency. Develop a clear, mutual understanding of what to expect of your psychiatrist and vice versa.

Reliably keeping appointments increases the chances of a successful outcome. As actor/director Woody Allen said, "The secret of success is showing up." Finding the right person for you is worth the time and effort spent in the search.

Don't be discouraged if you call a prospective psychiatrist only to find out that his or her practice is full or is no longer a provider with your insurance company. In the former situation, try what Julie did (see Chapter 6) and see if you can be placed on a waiting list and/or ask if the psychiatrist can suggest an available colleague. You may need to call your insurance company again for additional names or check your insurer's Internet site for a list of contracted psychiatrists.

8

Finding the Best Hospital and Emergency Room

A Tale of Success

James B is a fifty-four-year-old married engineer with three teenage daughters; they live in a midwestern city. James was grieving the death from heart attacks of his older brother and father seven years earlier. He was conscientious about all aspects of his life, especially his health and the welfare of his family. He was also conscientious about regular visits to his family physician and cardiologist. He exercised regularly and watched his diet.

Although he had received a clean bill of health from his doctors, he acknowledged his risk of succumbing to a heart attack and was concerned about staying healthy for the sake of his wife and his daughters, who were planning to go to college.

James had frank discussions with his cardiologist, not only about how to avoid risk factors for heart disease but also about which nearby hospitals were best equipped to treat heart patients. He and his devoted wife (who also was his health care advocate and had power of attorney for making medical decisions were he to become incapacitated) frankly discussed what they would do if James had a heart attack. He and his wife separately kept a list of all his medications, his recent EKGs, and the telephone numbers of the nearby ambulance service and the local hospital, which was accredited by the Joint Commission on Accreditation of Healthcare Organizations (JCAHO). They periodically made certain that the nearby hospital accepted his insurance.

They did not allow their concern about his risk for heart disease to disrupt their normal lives. Five years later, he was in good health. His children were in college and he and his wife were planning extended vacations. But they still maintained their preparedness should fate deal them a bad hand.

A Tale of Woe

Although several older family members had died of a stroke, Mrs. Smith, a fifty-year-old married high school physical education and nutrition teacher, always enjoyed good health but rarely visited her doctor. The subject of risk factors for stroke was never discussed with her husband or her physician. She avoided thinking about her hypertension and unhealthy diet – two common risk factors for a stroke. She didn't keep a list on hand of her medications. When the school district changed to a different health care insurer, which necessitated a change to a new physician, she put off finding one.

She awoke one morning with weakness on the right side of her body and slurred speech. Her husband called 911, and the emergency medics took her to the closest hospital. Neither she nor her husband notified the emergency room in advance, only to learn that her new insurance plan necessitated transfer to another hospital. It was not a JCAHO-accredited hospital, nor did it have a specialized stroke program.

Because Mrs. Smith had never found a new primary care physician (pcp), the emergency room staff had to waste precious time contacting her former physician to learn essential medical information. She died five days later of a hospital-acquired infection.

The moral of these two stories illustrates the importance of realistically accepting your vulnerability to a serious illness, reducing risk factors that may have adversely affected other family members, and being a proactive, conscientious, responsible patient. Your life and the lives of those you love may depend on it.

Finding the Best Hospital

The best time to decide on what emergency room (ER) or hospital to go to is when you are well, are not denying your vulnerability to a serious health problem, and aren't leaving the choice of ER to chance or to the ambulance driver. If you live in an average size city, you probably have several choices of ERs and hospitals besides the one closest to you. If your medical problem is serious, the major decision is what hospital is most capable of treating your particular medical, surgical, or psychiatric condition. Choosing the best hospital can make the difference between recovery or its opposite. Finding answers to the following questions ahead of time will prepare you if misfortune strikes.

1. Is the hospital and its emergency room accredited by JCAHO? Accredited facilities are most likely to have the best physicians specialized in emergency medicine and state-of-the-art medical equipment. Furthermore, if it is determined in the ER that you require hospitalization, you have a good chance of being admitted to the same hospital. One can check on a hospital's accreditation status via www.qualitycheck.org.

2. Does the hospital have specialists who treat your particular medical, surgical, or psychiatric problem?

3. Will your insurance pay for treatment at that particular hospital?

4. Will your pcp treat you at the hospital or, as in many large cities, does the hospital have full-time hospitalists (who treat sicker patients) and also intensivists (who are specially trained to treat critically ill patients in intensive care units)?

5. Is the hospital a teaching hospital affiliated with a medical school? These hospitals have medical students and residents closely supervised by experienced attending physicians with medical school appointments. On the negative side, teaching hospitals can be more burdensome on patients because multiple team members are questioning and examining you daily. Especially around July of every year, when a new crop of first-year resident physicians begins their training, less experienced trainees are involved in your care.

Finding the Best Emergency Room

Assuming that you've accepted that you are not invincible but vulnerable--like all other mortals--to a medical illness, there are a number of ways to decide, in advance, what emergency room is preferable. Important issues to consider:

1. Ask your pcp or friends who work in the medical field which ER they would choose.

2. Will your insurance company pay for that particular ER?

3. Is your pcp on staff at that hospital?

4. It may be prudent to go to the nearest ER if time is essential--for example, if you have a life-threatening illness such as a heart attack or a stroke.

5. Find out in advance the closest ER that specializes in trauma because such ERs have the most expertise in handling serious accidents. If the best trauma center is a

little farther from you, it may be worth the longer ride by ambulance.

6. For minor medical problems, consider a twenty-four-hour-a-day urgent care clinic near you. Getting in and out is faster and far less expensive than going to an ER. Well before an unexpected emergency, talk over all these factors with your spouse, partner, or health care advocate so you are both prepared to make the best decision.

For the more diligent consumer of ER services, you may (far in advance of needing such services) call the nurse manager of potential ERs to find out the ranking of that ER. Rankings range from 1 to 3, with 3 being the highest, indicating that they have advanced technological equipment and specialists either in attendance or who can be called in. You may also want to know the average wait time before the ER's physician sees patients because it can often take hours.

Remain As Calm and Collected As Possible

It's normal and natural to feel nervous and anxious when experiencing an acute medical problem – another reason to plan in advance to go to the best ER and hospital should a medical emergency occur. Have a family member, a friend, or your health care advocate notify the ER about your symptoms in advance of your arrival and accompany you to the ER to help explain your current symptoms, medications, past health problems, allergies, et cetera. Bring a copy of your health care profile, your insurance cards, and a list of current medications. The ER can therefore be better prepared when you arrive. You and your health care advocate or the person accompanying you to the ER, should bring two documents--your advance directive and your durable power of attorney for health care decisions--in case the person having that responsibility needs to make health care decisions on your behalf.

Some hospitals provide you with a health care advocate if you do not have one. You can request one upon entering the emergency room or hospital.

What to Do Before Going to the ER

1. If you are seriously ill, call or have someone call 911 for an ambulance. Don't drive yourself if you are seriously ill.

2. Call or ask your health care advocate to call your pcp and (a) explain your symptoms, (b) ask your pcp to contact the ER, and (c) also ask your pcp if he or she can meet you at the ER.

3. Ask someone (ideally your health care advocate or family member) to call your insurance company because some require advance notification if you use an ambulance service or go to an ER.

4. Pack a small suitcase with essential clothes, toiletries, your health care profile, any medications, and your personal telephone directory in case you are admitted to the hospital.

After Arriving at the ER

1. You, a family member, or your health care advocate should explain to the triage nurse, in a clear and concise manner, your main symptoms and problems so the nurse can determine the seriousness of your condition. Give the nurse your health care profile. All this information can help the triage nurse expedite the next step in diagnosing and treating your condition.

2. If you think you are having a serious, potentially fatal medical illness, you or your health care advocate can tell

the nurse or the physician assistant that you want to see the ER's attending physician.

3. Expect to feel scared and frightened, not only because of your symptoms and not knowing your diagnosis, but also because most busy emergency rooms are noisy and brightly lit. You may see patients more critically ill than you. Don't make yourself more upset by taking personally what you may perceive to be some negative remarks by an ER staff member about another patient. Doctors and nurses are under considerable stress and sometimes use humor to help them cope.

4. Despite these stresses, try to maintain trust and faith in the medical team, and be cooperative with them. It's expected that you and your health care advocate will have questions to ask. Depending on your degree of anxiety, you may even feel tempted to refuse diagnostic tests, medication, and hospitalization or, worse, request to be discharged from the ER against medical advice. This may lead to worsening of your medical problem. Your health care advocate may understand your situation more rationally and will advise you to cooperate.

9

Preparing for Surgery

Be Inquisitive and Informed

D on't be shy about asking important questions of the surgeon and members of your health care team. You may have grown up in an era when you were taught to act reverently and submissively with the doctor in his long white coat. Some surgeons look and behave in an authoritative manner, which may make you feel intimidated and uncertain whether or not you are acting respectfully if you ask questions. You may even feel that your questions will be perceived as a sign of disrespect, but this is not the case. Your health care team wants and expects you to be fully informed before you agree to have surgery so that you are prepared for what to expect before, during, and after surgery.

Another reason you may avoid asking questions is fear of finding out disturbing information you would prefer not to know. You can ask your health care advocate to ask questions on your behalf. One way of overcoming your hesitation about asking questions is just by forging ahead. You will benefit from being a conscientious, fully informed patient.

Before and during your stay in the hospital, write down your questions and include additional concerns as they come to mind. It's normal and natural to experience some anxiety when the physician in an academic teaching hospital enters your room, often accompanied by an entourage of residents and medical students. Nervousness may make you forget some important questions. This is when your list comes in handy. The principal surgeon may not have time to answer all your questions, but members of his or her team will.

Here are some examples of the types of questions you are fully entitled to ask. You, your family, and health care advocate may think of others.

1. What are the risks and benefits of having this surgery?

2. Are there alternative treatments for my condition other than surgery?

3. Are there newer ways to perform the surgery that are less invasive?

4. What can I do to best prepare for surgery?

5. Which of my medicines should I take on the days and the evening before surgery?

6. How long might I need to stay in the hospital after the surgery?

7. What kinds of complications are most frequent, and what is done to treat them?

8. What kind of anesthesia will be best for me, and are there alternatives that entail less risk?

9. How soon after surgery can I get out of bed and walk around?

10. How much pain may I expect after surgery and what painkillers will I receive?

11. After I return home, who should I call about unexpected complications?

For elective surgery (which is planned ahead of time) rather than emergency surgery, you and/or your advocate should make an appointment early on with the hospital business office to discuss the expected approximate costs of your hospitalization—specifically, what expenses will be paid by your insurance company and what you will be expected to pay. Expect separate bills from the hospital, surgeon, anesthesiologist, X-ray department, and others. Also discuss this with your insurance company. For emergency surgery, these issues can be handled after the fact by you and/or your health care advocate.

Some studies have suggested that the day and time that you are admitted to the hospital for surgery can influence your chances for a good outcome. For example, people admitted to a hospital for elective (non-emergent) surgery on holidays or have anesthesia late in the afternoon rather than in the morning are less likely to have good outcomes and more likely to have complications. This is not to suggest, however, that--should you require emergency surgery on a holiday--you stay home and wait until a weekday morning.

Choosing the Best Surgeon

You want to select a very well trained, experienced surgeon specialized in the operation that you are having, especially if it's a technically difficult procedure. You're unlikely to have a long-term, ongoing relationship with the surgeon, so bedside manner is of less importance than his or her technical skill. As an analogy, you want a car mechanic who can fix your transmission correctly the first time; his or her interpersonal manner is less important.

Finding an excellent surgeon is not unlike finding the best specialist for a complicated medical or mental health problem. The search begins by asking your primary care physician (pcp) for recommendations, but you'll need to be a keen investigator to determine whether he or she is the best surgeon for your particular operation, as illustrated by the following example.

My mentor, the director of the state mental health institute in Chicago where I worked, developed coronary artery disease and needed to have cardiac bypass surgery. Fortunately, he knew the best cardiac surgeons at the nearby academic medical center. Because he was very bright and intuitive, his investigative talents helped him to not only find the best heart surgeon but also the one most experienced in bypassing the left anterior coronary artery. He felt calm and confidant about his upcoming surgery, which contributed to his smooth recovery. When I visited him in the hospital, he gave me a reassuring wink about having chosen the right surgeon.

Finding one of the best surgeons sometimes calls for an Internet search. You want to find a surgeon who is Board certified in the specialty for your particular surgery, for example, a Board-certified cardiovascular surgeon if you require heart surgery. Is your prospective surgeon a fellow of the American College of Surgeons (ACS), indicated by the letters FACS after his or her name? To find this out, ask his or her receptionist or nurse, or visit www.facs.org and enter the surgeon's name, or call 800-621-4111 and find names of fellows of the ACS. Some managed care plans do not permit you to find your own surgeon, so you need to contact your insurance company for the names of surgeons who are contracted providers.

If you want to find one of the very best surgeons in the country involved in the most advanced cutting-edge research in the technique specific to your condition, go to www.pubmed.gov. After entering the name of the particular surgical technique (such as cardiac bypass surgery), make note of repeatedly named authors of published papers. These are likely to be among the most experienced researchers and practicing surgeons. While carrying out this search, you may learn of some recent surgical techniques that are less invasive and have better outcomes than previous approaches.

You can then share what you've learned with your pcp and ask his or her opinion about contacting one of these surgeons to consult on your case. If your family, work, other responsibilities, and financial situation permit, you may consider traveling for an appointment to the city where the surgeon practices. Keep in mind that "new " surgical technique doesn't always mean "better," but getting a second opinion may help you feel more secure in your decision.

If you want additional opinions, consider asking a surgical nurse or an anesthesiologist at the hospital where you are contemplating surgery what surgeon they would choose were they to need your particular surgery.

Choosing the Best Hospital

If the surgeon you have selected operates at only one or two hospitals, that's where you'll have your operation. However, the quality of the hospital is equally important as the surgeon, so you want a JCAHO-accredited hospital. If the operation is complicated, selecting a large teaching hospital assures you of very experienced staff who can effectively deal with postoperative complications, which can be more worrisome than the actual surgery.

To be assured you'll be treated at a high-quality hospital, go to www.JCAHO.org or www.jointcommission.org and enter the name of the hospital to see if it is accredited, to confirm that the hospital has complied with the Joint Commission National Patient Safety goals and to substantiate that the surgeon has performed your specific operation many, many times. Studies have shown that patients have better outcomes if their particular type of surgery is done at a hospital that has carried out a great number of such surgeries.

Pre-Surgery Visit with Your Surgeon and Anesthesiologist

You may have a preliminary discussion with the surgeon prior to hospitalization. Patients are usually hospitalized a day or two before an elective (non-emergent) surgery. The day before surgery, expect visits from the surgeon, his or her associate surgeon, and the anesthesiologist. It is important to be frank and honest. For example, if you have an alcohol or drug abuse problem, be clear about this to both the surgeon and the anesthesiologist because addicted persons can experience life-threatening withdrawal symptoms postoperatively. Likewise, patients who have a long-term dependency on pain medications, such as hydrocodone, oxycodone, or meperidine, may have built up a tolerance to pain medications and therefore may require higher doses following surgery. If pain medication is abruptly stopped, dangerous withdrawal symptoms may develop.

The anesthesiologist will want to know whether you recall having had a bad reaction to anesthesia you had in the past (although you may not remember this), what medications you are currently taking, if you have drug allergies, and your opinion about your pain threshold. If given a choice, consider selecting the type of anesthesia with the least likelihood of complications.

The surgeon and anesthesiologist will explain all the risks and benefits associated with your surgery and ask that you sign a consent form acknowledging your understanding and willingness to undergo the anesthesia and surgery. This gives you (and your advocate, if present) another opportunity to ask questions.

You can ask the anesthesiologist if he or she or a nurse anesthetist will administer the anesthesia, and, likewise, if the surgeon or a resident in training will perform or only assist the attending surgeon. It's appropriate to make your preferences known. Most patients prefer the most experienced surgeon and anesthesiologist rather than a resident in training.

If you are admitted to a hospital in an emergency and you lack the mental capacity to make an informed decision and sign a consent form, the hospital will try to obtain consent from a responsible family member. If you have a health care proxy for making medical decisions on your behalf if you are incapacitated, the surgeon or hospital representative will try to obtain that person's consent. If emergency surgery is required to save your life, and consents can not be obtained, the surgeon and hospital will proceed in your best interest.

Dealing with Pain

Even if you pride yourself on having a high pain threshold, don't feel you have to prove it to yourself or others. Make certain that you leave the hospital or outpatient surgical center with a sufficient amount of pain medication best suited to you. If you are allergic to a particular type of pain medication, remind your physician. It's best to use pain medication for as short a period as possible because chronic use runs the risk of psychological or physical dependency and development of tolerance (needing higher doses for pain relief). For mild to moderate pain, aspirin or non-steroidal anti-inflammatory drugs (NSAIDs) such as ibuprofen are usually sufficient. NSAIDs also reduce swelling. It's best to take them with food because they can cause irritation and bleeding of the stomach as well as nausea, and can interfere with blood clotting.

For severe pain, opiods such as oxycodone, codeine, meperidine, or morphine are often prescribed. It's preferable to use them for short periods unless your doctor recommends one of them for severe chronic pain and its use can be carefully monitored by your doctor. Side effects include constipation, nausea, drowsiness, and impaired coordination, respiration, and urination.

Hydromorphone is much stronger than morphine and is usually given intravenously for relieving moderate to severe pain. It is sometimes used in the recovery room after surgery.

10

What You Need to Know About Medications

A dvances in medical science, healthier lifestyles, and newer more effective medications have accounted for vastly increased life expectancy since the early 1900s. Better, safer medications instill in patients hope and faith in faster recovery from illness.

It is important to maintain faith and confidence in the prescribing physician and the medications you are taking. This is especially true because you don't often see or feel the effects, such as with cholesterol-lowering medication.

When pharmacies fill your prescription, it has become standard for them to give you a long list of potential side effects. And the Internet is replete with additional warnings and safeguards you want to be familiar with. But be mindful that pharmaceutical companies are required to list every suspected side effect that occurs during their clinical trials before medications are approved by the Food and Drug Administration (FDA) and come to market. Try not to be overly vigilant, and avoid allowing your understandable anxiety about taking a new medication to make you over-interpret some unrelated physical discomfort as evidence of a side effect. When in doubt, though, call your physician.

Having faith and confidence in your medications and your prescribing physician facilitates your recovery, yet the conscientious patient needs to be mindful not only of the potential benefits of medications but also the risk of side effects, drug-drug interactions, and common mistakes in taking medications. In other words, find a comfortable balance between trust and vigilance.

This chapter reviews common problems associated with taking medications, ways of avoiding errors, questions to ask your prescribing doctor, ways of avoiding side effects, advantages of using different types of pharmacies and using your pharmacist as your ally, special considerations regarding the elderly, ways to reduce costs, and how to obtain medication if you don't have health insurance.

Common Problems

If medications are ineffective, it is often because patients do not take them properly, discontinue them prematurely, or do not take them at all. It is estimated that only half of all prescribed medications are taken properly. Improper use of medications results in more than a million Americans becoming seriously ill each year. Common causes of medication mishaps include taking the wrong medication and the wrong dose, pharmacy errors, medication side effects (adverse reactions), and drug-drug interactions.

Avoiding Medication Errors

As a conscientious patient, do not assume that all your health care providers regularly share with one another information about your medications and changes in your health status. You, and sometimes with the assistance of your health care advocate, need to be active communicators with all your health care professionals.

For example, you may be under the care of several physicians and other health care professionals who are unaware of medications prescribed by others. So keep on your person at all times an updated list of all your current prescribed medications, over-the-counter medications and herbal remedies, a list of drug allergies and other allergies, and your medical/psychiatric diagnoses. Give your updated lists of all your medications at each visit to all your health care professionals. Keeping your up-to-date list in your wallet or purse will be invaluable if you find yourself in an emergency room.

Additional Safeguards

1. Have your prescriptions filled and take medications reliably. One-third of prescriptions in the United States never get filled.

2. Keep your medications in the original bottles rather than combining them in a single bottle because many look alike.

3. If you are taking several medications daily, use a plastic pill dispenser available at any pharmacy to remind you to take your medications at the right time and as a reminder of whether or not you have taken them.

4. When picking up your medications at the pharmacy, check that your name, the name of the medication, the number of pills, the dosage, and the labels are correct, especially if you are using a busy large retail pharmacy. I often learn from my patients that they were given an insufficient number of pills.

5. Keep an extra week's supply of all your pills in a safe place in case you lose some or the mail-order service is late in delivering them.

6. Don't break or crush your pills or capsules because their effectiveness may be diminished. If uncertain, read the directions that came with the pills, or call your pharmacist or doctor.

7. Resist pressure from a friend or family member to share your pills with them because it is risky, and you will be practicing medicine without a license.

8. Take pain medication, such as opiods like oxycodon, at the times recommended by your physician. Under his or her supervision, cooperate in reducing their use to avoid the risk of becoming psychologically or physically dependent on them.

9. Don't abruptly stop medicine you have been taking a long or even a short period of time without first discussing it with your doctor. Some medications need to be slowly tapered under medical supervision before discontinuation.

10. When traveling, especially air travel, keep your medications on your person at all times in case your luggage is lost.

11. Keep medications in a dry, cool place rather than a hot, humid bathroom cabinet, where moisture and heat can reduce their effectiveness.

12. Before undergoing a procedure requiring insertion of dyes or radioactive material, remind the attending staff of any allergies you have.

13. Although most medications are effective for weeks or months past the expiration date noted on the bottle, throw away outdated medications no longer used to avoid using inactive medications or the risk of someone else using them.

14. Keep a careful daily record of the names of medications and the time they are taken to ensure you have not missed a dose. Record suspected side effects. Show your medication record to your doctors and other health care

professionals so they can monitor your compliance and possible side effects.

15. Call your physician in ample time before you run out of your medication to make certain you have an adequate supply.

Do Some Research Before Visiting Your Physician

If you suspect that your physician is too busy to know whether there are less costly brand-name or generic medications available, then you and/or your health care advocate can do some research and planning before visiting your physician. If you have a common medical problem such as diabetes, hypertension, or depression, it's almost certain that there are generic or older brand-name medications that may be equally effective but much less expensive.

If you know your diagnosis, before visiting your doctor call your pharmacist with your prescription drug insurance card in hand and find out what commonly used drugs are available to treat your condition, what drugs are partly or entirely covered by your insurance, and if there are generic alternatives that are equally effective but much less costly. You can also search the Internet.

With this information in hand, when you visit your physician, before he or she writes a prescription for a brand-name medication, ask whether there is a less expensive but equally effective generic medication. Also, mention the one or two less expensive brand-name and generic medications you learned about from your pharmacist or on the Internet. Don't be embarrassed to ask for a less expensive medication because physicians are sensitive to the financial strain that patients experience, especially during hard economic times.

If you have not succeeded in obtaining a prescription from your physician for a reasonably priced medication and later discover at the pharmacy that the prescription is not covered or is insufficiently covered by your insurance and will cost hundreds of dollars per month, ask your pharmacist to call your physician to inquire about a generic equivalent or a less expensive brand-name medication.

Questions to Ask Your Doctor When Given a New Prescription

Consider asking some of the following questions when given a new prescription. Your physician will respect your wish to be fully informed and knowledgeable. Some pertinent questions include:

1. What illness is this medication being used to treat?

2. At what time intervals do I take the medication, and do I take it with or without food?

3. Does this new medication replace any pills I'm currently taking?

4. How long should I take the medication? Don't make the mistake of stopping the medication as soon as symptoms improve because the illness and its symptoms may return. If uncertain, check with your physician.

5. What are any potential side effects, and how common are they?

6. How safe is it to take this medication with my other medications, including herbal remedies and organic supplements?

7. Is this new medication and are my other medications safe to take with alcohol and recreational drugs such as marijuana? When the physician asks how much you drink and use recreational drugs, be honest because of the natural tendency to deny or minimize their use, with potentially dire consequences.

8. Are there any activities I should avoid? (For example, certain tranquilizers can make your skin sensitive to sun exposure.)

9. Will you write for prescription refills or do I need to contact you?

10. If your physician has good reasons for prescribing the more expensive brand-name medication because it is more effective or there is no generic equivalent, and the brand-name medication is not covered by your insurance, the doctor's office may need to call the prescription benefit department of your insurance company (the phone number is sometimes on the back of your insurance card) to have a prior authorization form faxed to the doctor's office. Some physician offices have ready access to these prior authorization forms. However, if your physician is in solo practice without office staff, he or she may ask you to call the prescription department of your insurance company to have the authorization form faxed to his or her office. Your physician then explains why it is imperative for you to have the brand-name medication. The authorization form is faxed from the doctor's office to the insurance company. If the request is approved, the insurance company notifies you and your physician and you can then obtain the medication at a reasonable cost.

Avoiding Side Effects

There are three main safeguards against the risk of medication side effects and drug-drug interactions. The safeguards are your physician, your pharmacist, and, most importantly, *you*, the conscientious patient.

Your doctor keeps a record of all your medications. Many physicians have hand-held computers on which they can check about drug-drug interactions. Keep your doctor in the information loop by keeping him or her informed about any over-the-counter medications that you take and medications prescribed by all your other doctors.

Another safeguard is your local pharmacist, whose computer system checks your new prescription with the medications you are currently taking. The pharmacist can inform you about possible side effects, drug-drug interactions, and unnecessary duplication with other medications you may be taking for the same illness. Inform your doctor and obtain advice about what to do. Also consider using the same pharmacy each time in order to develop a cooperative relationship with your pharmacist, who may take a special interest in your welfare and safeguard you against these potential problems.

What to Know About Drug-Drug Interactions

The risk of medication side effects has increased because of increasing life expectancy, the greater use of multiple medications and over-the-counter meds, and pressure by patients on physicians to prescribe drugs advertised on TV. Also, there may be genetic factors that influence how you absorb, metabolize, and respond to drugs, and the ability of your liver and kidneys to metabolize and excrete them. The ever-increasing number of new medications manufactured by pharmaceutical companies also contributes to the risk of side effects.

Half of all adults in the United States take two or more medications a day, and it is not unusual for persons over age seventy to be taking six or more different medications, thus increasing the risk for side effects and drug-drug interactions. The following is just a sampling of common drug-drug interactions to be mindful of.

Medication	Interacts with	Increases risk of
Aspirin	Non-steroidal anti-inflammatory drugs (NSAIDs) such as ibuprofen	Stomach irritation and bleeding
SSRI antidepressants such as paroxetine and fluoxetine or tricyclic antidepressants such as amitriptyline and imipramine	St.-John's-wort (an over-the-counter medication believed by some to improve mild depression but has properties that inhibit the enzyme monoamine oxidase)	Hypertension, nervousness, confusion
SSRI antidepressants	Tricyclic antidepressants (such as amitriptyline, imipramine, nortriptyline, desipramine)	Lowered blood pressure, confusion, constipation, urinary retention, dry mouth. Combining these medications increases the blood level of tricyclic antidepressant. Need to monitor the blood level of the tricyclic antidepressant
Benzodiazepines (anti-anxiety drugs such as lorazepam, diazepam, chlordiazepoxide)	Alcohol, barbiturates	Balance issues, drowsiness, forgetfulness
Opiates, such as oxycodone, oxycotin	Benzodiazepines, alcohol	Drowsiness, difficulty breathing, psychological and physical dependency

Medication	Interacts with	Increases risk of
Cholesterol-lowering drugs (such as lovastatin, simvastatin)	Grapefruit or grapefruit juice	Can cause muscle damage
Some antibiotics and heart drugs	Grapefruit or grapefruit juice	Can increase the blood levels of the antibiotic and heart drugs, causing side effects
Antibiotic Erythromycin	Anticonvulsant drugs such as carbamazepine	Increased blood levels of anticonvulsant, causing drowsiness and gait disturbance
Erythromycin	Statin drugs used to lower blood cholesterol	Increased risk of muscle soreness and damage

Three Major Types of Pharmacies

Advantages of a Small Neighborhood Pharmacy

There are advantages to using a small neighborhood pharmacy. You can establish a good, long-term working relationship with your pharmacist, and you'll benefit from personal service, short waiting lines, and infrequent staff turnover. And small pharmacies often have the same advantages of chain pharmacies:

1. They have a record of all the prescriptions you have filled in the past, including those from your other doctors.

2. They may have a computer system that can detect potential drug-drug interactions.

3. They are knowledgeable about medication side effects.

4. They know when to call your doctor with questions about your prescriptions.

5. They may be able to accept prescriptions that are electronically sent from your doctor's office, reducing errors from misread handwritten prescriptions.

If you are using your neighborhood pharmacy and value one or two particular pharmacists, learn their schedules so you can bring in prescriptions or questions when they are on duty.

Advantages of a Large Countrywide Pharmacy

There are also advantages to using a large countrywide pharmacy. Mega pharmacies are more technologically organized, have larger supplies of various medications, and sometimes are less expensive. Some are open twenty-four hours a day, seven days a week. If you travel frequently and run out of medications while you're away, a big chain pharmacy's computer system can communicate with the branch pharmacy near your home to verify who you are and contact your physician to get approval for a supply of medication to last until your next office visit. Large pharmacy chains have more locations, so you have easier access to them. The disadvantages of mega pharmacies are similar to those of large discount stores, including impersonal service, longer waiting lines, and frequent staff turnover.

Mail-Order Pharmacy

A third option is to use a mail-order pharmacy, which is usually less expensive and will sometimes send reminder letters or calls when your medication requires a refill. If you know you will be taking certain medications over the long term and don't require the personal attention of a neighborhood pharmacy, a mail-order pharmacy may be adequate for your needs. Notify the mail-order service weeks before your supply of medications runs low because mail delivery can be slow during holidays and other times. If you know you will need a certain medication for a long time, it may be possible, depending on your insurance company's policy, to buy a three-month or longer supply from your mail-order company. Local pharmacies can do this as well.

Special Considerations Regarding the Elderly

Elderly patients may benefit from being under the care of a physician specializing in geriatrics because of the complicated nature of their multiple problems and the greater need for coordinated care.

The likelihood of side effects increases with the greater number of medications taken. Studies at large universities found that over 20 percent of older patients were taking medications with a high potential for side effects. Those older than sixty-five are often taking five or more prescription medications (in addition to herbal remedies and over-the-counter medications), so there is a greater likelihood for side effects and drug-drug interactions. Elderly persons metabolize and excrete drugs more slowly and are prone to developing high blood levels of certain drugs; an example is long-half-life benzodiazepines such as diazepam and chlordiazepoxide. Overuse of benzodiazepines, especially with the elderly, can contribute to balance issues and falling, memory problems, and drowsiness.

In addition, the elderly may be more prone to medication errors because of visual, hearing, and cognitive impairment and concomitant alcohol and drug abuse. One or a combination of these factors can impair judgment. For example, an older person may awaken in the middle of the night not remembering whether he or she had taken a sleep medication, and then mistakenly take more--with dire consequences.

These risks point to the need for a pill dispenser so a daily or weekly supply of pills can be placed in the appropriate compartment. The very frail, impaired, elderly person can benefit from a dependable health care advocate, and sometimes from a part-time or twenty-four-hour-a-day caregiver who can oversee and monitor dispensing of pills, ensure attendance at physician appointments, and other aspects of health care.

The mismanagement of my seventy-eight-year-old Aunt Susan's medical care, discussed in the introduction of this book, is a distressing example of what can happen when coordination of treatment is lacking. She was seeing several doctors who did not communicate with one another. Her psychiatrist prescribed amitriplyline for depression and quetiapine – a major tranquilizer – for insomnia and nervousness. Her internist, not knowing the other medications she was taking, prescribed a long-acting benzodiazepine for insomnia. Within a week, she became confused, over-sedated, constipated, and agitated and was found wandering aimlessly around her neighborhood. Taken to the emergency room, she was diagnosed as having drug-induced delirium from the combined side effects of her medications. Her medications were discontinued and her confusion resolved.

Conscientious Patients Can Save on Drug Costs

Insurance companies have shifted more of the financial burden onto you – the consumer – in the form of higher co-pays and deductibles. Patients with multiple illnesses can pay thousands of dollars each year for prescription drugs. Many seriously ill patients with limited financial means are forced to choose between the necessities of life (food, clothing, and shelter) or the medications necessary for their survival.

After a pharmaceutical company's brand-name medication has been on the market for a certain number of years (usually twelve to fourteen years), other companies can make generic drugs that are often (but unfortunately not always) as effective as the brand-name drug. This may not be a serious concern for generic drugs manufactured in the United States because the Federal Drug Administration (FDA) provides oversight. But be careful of generic drugs manufactured in Asia, Mexico, and other regions of the world where oversight and quality can be deficient. Also, unscrupulous companies make counterfeit drugs that are worthless.

Sometimes pharmaceutical companies will come out with a once-daily new version of the same medication that is usually taken two or three times daily. The once-daily new variant of the same medication may be much more expensive but not more effective than the multiple-dose variety, so consider the latter.

Sometimes you pay as much for a high-dosage pill as for a lower-dose pill. Ask your physician or pharmacist whether the higher-dose pill, which costs the same, would have the same effectiveness if you were to divide it with a pill cutter.

If you want your physician to write a prescription for a brand-name medication, make certain that the "no substitution" box is checked on the prescription.

You can sometimes save substantially by buying medications from Canada. Check these Internet sites: www.discountdrugsfromcanada.com or call 516-731-1500, www.canadianpharmacy.com, and www.Jandrugs.com.

If You Don't Have Prescription Drug Insurance

One alternative is to go to the Internet site Consumer Reports Best Buy Drugs (www.crbestbuydrugs.org), which provides a list of reasonably priced drugs for various common ailments. With this information, you or the pharmacist can call your physician to consider the lower-cost medications. Big discount department stores such as Walmart, Target, and Costco have a great variety of generic drugs that cost about $4 for a one-month supply.

Buying Medications on the Internet

Be cautious when buying medications on the Internet because some unscrupulous companies sell counterfeit pills; many are manufactured outside the United States. Also, be wary of sites that do not require a prescription, especially for narcotic drugs. Or you may want to avoid buying any drugs on the Internet simply because it can be very risky.

Verify that the Internet company is legitimate and has a person you can talk to on the phone. Also, confirm that the Internet company is certified by the Verified Internet Pharmacy Practice Site (VIPPS), which means it has met standards set by the National Association of Boards of Pharmacy. If you do not see the VIPPS seal and are suspicious, you can check the National Associations' Board at www.nabp.net/vipps/intro.asp to verify that the Internet pharmacy is licensed and in good standing.

If You Have Medicare Without Part D

Medicare offers a discount program for those with Medicare Parts A and B but not Part D (the drug benefit) and without a secondary insurance. The program covers prescription medication for those earning less than $12,570 a year (or $16,863 for a married couple). Medicare's discount card costs $30 annually and provides a considerable discount on prescription drugs. For information, call 1-800-MEDICARE, or check www.medicare.gov.

Sample Drugs from Your Physician's Office

Another strategy to reduce the cost of expensive brand-name medication is to ask your physician if he or she has samples that you can try before investing in a one-month or more supply. Keep in mind that the samples are brand name rather than generic drugs, so when you eventually need to purchase them and your insurance doesn't cover part of the cost, it can be very expensive.

Samples may help save you considerable money but only if you will need this medication for a short time because your physician may have a limited supply that is dependent on the ability of the pharmaceutical representative to provide additional samples. Once generic equivalents of the brand-name medication become available, your physician may no longer be able to obtain samples of the brand-name medication. Ask your physician what you can expect if you rely on samples. If the physician's supply of sample brand-name medication is limited and unreliable and/or you will need this medication for weeks or months, you may want to use one of the other strategies described in this chapter.

What If You Need an Expensive Medication

If you have a serious, rare ailment that requires an expensive brand-name medication because there are no inexpensive alternatives, there are prescription assistance programs run by private companies and foundations to help lower costs. Go to the Internet site Prescription Drug Assistance Programs-- Consumer Reports; then go to "Partnership for Prescription Assistance," which offers a guide for choosing the best program. You can type in the name of the drug you need and/or the state in which you live.

If you do not have prescription insurance, need an expensive medication, and have a low yearly income, contact Together Rx Access, which offers discounts on more than 275 drugs. Call 1-800-444-4106, or go to www.trxaccess.com.

Many pharmaceutical companies offer discounts on their brand-name drugs for low-income individuals, such as the Pfizer PFriends Program (1-866-706-2400, or go to www.pfizerhelpfulanswers.com). Janssen Pharmaceuticals has a patient assistance program (1-800-652-6227, or www.janssen.com). Find out the company that manufactures the medication you need, enter the name on your Internet browser screen, and find out if the company offers a similar drug discount program.

Consumer Ingenuity and Persistence

Alice is a well-respected and valued surgical nursing supervisor for four units at a university medical center in the

Midwest. She periodically became emotionally crippled by a treatment-resistant depression that barely enabled her to get out of bed in the morning. All other approaches to her severe depression had been tried. Her antidepressant was effective only if she took it along with an "off label" augmenting mood-enhancing drug that was not approved by the FDA for depression but only for certain sleep disorders.

The off label drug wasn't approved by her insurance company despite several authorization requests by her psychiatrist along with research articles supporting its effectiveness. She could not afford the medication, which cost more than $1,000 per month.

Alice did some investigating of her own and located the name and telephone number of the physician head of her insurance company's prescription drug department. Tactfully but assertively, she explained the dire circumstances affecting her personal life, her career, and the functioning of the surgical units she supervised if the insurance company would not pay for the mood-enhancing drug. She implied that she was so desperate that she would have an attorney start a lawsuit against the insurance company. As a result, her request was approved within minutes, enabling her to continue her successful career.

Being a Smart Purchaser of Prescription Drug Insurance – Now and Under the Affordable Care Act (ACA)

Under the ACA, if you are not covered by Medicare, Medicaid, the Veterans Administration (VA), your employer, or under your parents' insurance, you will be able to purchase medical and prescription drug insurance on an insurance exchange. The following is an approximation, not a certainty, of how this will work under the ACA. It is planned that this exchange will list all available insurance policies, dividing them into a hierarchy of levels from "silver" to "gold" to "platinum." Keep in mind that only some of these policies will cover prescription drugs. Compare these different policies carefully. Don't assume that because two policies are both "gold" that they offer similar prescription drug coverage.

It may be less expensive to first choose a medical insurance plan (for hospital and doctor visits), then select a separate prescription drug policy that covers the drugs that you and your family will be using over the long term. Make a list of all the drugs that you and family members are currently taking and may use in the future. Then check to see which prescription plan includes the drugs you will need.

Using Medicare as an example of how to choose a prescription drug plan, if you are about to select a Part D prescription plan--such as AARP's United Health Care Plan or Humana--refer to your list of medications and see which prescription plan covers most if not all of them. Call your pharmacist or independent insurance agent to assist you in deciding the best prescription drug insurance plan for you.

I am the first to admit that deciding on health and prescription drug insurance can be confusing, frustrating, and time-consuming. We may witness a change in the rules of the ACA as we get closer to the starting gate on January 1, 2014, especially when political partisanship continues attempting to make changes. So enlist the advice of your independent insurance agent, health care advocate, or a friend who works in the health care field to help you make important insurance decisions. Given the ever-increasing costs of health care in America, purchase the best, most inclusive insurance you can afford to protect you and your family from a devastating and costly illness.

11

Surviving Your Stay in the Hospital

A stay in the hospital is very stressful and evokes profound, unwelcome feelings of dependency and sometimes hopelessness. You may be in a weakened, susceptible state to begin with, and your anxiety level may be high. Stripped away is your sense of self--who you are as a person, reinforced by familiarity with your surroundings, the security of friends and family, and feeling control over your destiny. Familiar trappings such as your clothes, wallet, and personal belongings are stored away for you.

When you enter the hospital, you are expected to conform to a new, strange, and potentially bewildering environment. A white hospital gown is substituted for your clothes. You are expected to be passive, submissive to your care providers, and compliant with recommended tests and treatments. Meals and the scheduling of tests and procedures are out of your control. You may feel dependent on a system that is far from perfect. It's unsettling to know that about 98,000 hospitalized patients die yearly from hospital errors, and about twenty times that number (about 2 million patients) come down with a hospital-related infection, according to the Centers for Disease Control and Prevention.

What can you do to make your stay in the hospital safe and successful? Read on for advice on preparing for your stay in the hospital, avoiding the risks associated with hospitalization, what to do if you have a justifiable complaint about your stay in the hospital, how to handle questions about your bill, and preparing for a safe return home.

Preparing for Your Stay in the Hospital

It's worth repeating that it is advisable to select a hospital accredited by the Joint Commission on Accreditation of Healthcare Organizations (JCAHO), and to know in advance who will be responsible for coordinating all your care--whether it will be your primary care physician (pcp) or a specialist (for example, a surgeon) or a hospital-employed physician (hospitalist). The trend is for hospitals in large cities to use hospitalists, in which case the doctor with whom you are most familiar (such as your pcp) may not be your doctor in the hospital.

Your close family members and your health care advocate and all the health care professionals involved in your care in the hospital should know who is responsible for coordinating all your care, including approval of recommendations from consultants and coordinating tests and medications so errors are avoided. If you don't have a family member or a friend who can serve as your health care advocate, some hospitals can provide one, so ask beforehand.

It is sometimes up to you or your advocate to make certain that records from your pcp and your other physicians reach your hospital physician as quickly as possible. Bring to the hospital a copy of your health care directive and your durable power of attorney for health care decisions, which specify who would make medical decisions on your behalf should you lack the capacity to do so.

Have your health care advocate listen and take notes during physician visits, ask questions that you may have inadvertently forgotten, field questions from family and friends about your progress, and provide you with emotional support.

Your advocate does not require a medical or nursing background. You want someone who is reliable and organized and stays calm and rational in a crisis. A good advocate frees you up to concentrate on getting well, thus enabling you to have a shorter, safer hospital stay. Let all members of your health care team know who your advocate is and what role he or she is carrying out on your behalf.

If your hospitalization is an elective one (non-emergent and scheduled in advance), you have time to pack a small suitcase that includes your personal telephone directory, a small bottle of sanitizer (to supplement one given to you in the hospital), toiletries, a change of clothing, and perhaps your cell phone and some personal items, such as a family photograph. Jewelry, whether expensive or not, is better left at home. It can be a breeding place for infection and needs to be removed if special X-rays are needed. Bring a complete list of all your current medications and the actual pill bottles so the physician (who may be a hospitalist) and the nurses know exactly what you were taking before hospitalization. Bring all your insurance cards, including secondary insurance cards. Selectively notify your close family and friends (or have your advocate help) of where you are, and decide whether or not you want them to know about your health problem and whether or not you want them to visit you. It's best to limit visitors to a minimum so you can focus your energies on getting well and avoid catching a visitor's infection. Designate one family member or friend (who may be your advocate) to speak directly with your hospital doctor and other hospital staff, because it can be burdensome for them if several family members want answers to similar questions but then don't communicate with one another.

Avoiding the Risks of Hospitalization

To safeguard your stay in the hospital, you need to strike a fine balance between being the consummate diplomat and being a hypervigilant sleuth. You want to avoid being perceived by hospital staff members--who are dedicated to helping you--as cantankerous, mistrustful, and cranky.

Keep in mind that there is a nationwide shortage of nurses, so they often work long hours and are underappreciated. Hospitals often have to hire locum tenens (temporary) nurses from other cities or countries who work for short periods of time and are less familiar with hospital procedures. So it is to everyone's benefit for you, your family, and friends to act respectful and appreciative of the nurses' concern and professionalism. Write down the names of your nurses and attendants and any personal information they may share with you. Calling the people who care for you by name helps create good feelings among the hospital staff.

Avoiding Infections

One of the gravest risks of hospitalization, especially with long hospital stays, is a hospital-acquired infection. If you have an illness that reduces your body's natural defenses against infection (such as an autoimmune disease), you are more susceptible to a hospital-acquired infection. Bacterial, fungal, and viral infections can significantly complicate and prolong your hospital stay.

An important way to safeguard against a hospital-acquired infection is by choosing a JCAHO-accredited hospital that has passed rigorous tests, including inspections for cleanliness and sterile techniques. Safe hospitals have a multitude of sinks, soap, and hand-cleaning dispensers near every bedside.

One of the most crucial ways to safeguard against a hospital infection is frequently washing your hands and making certain that physicians, nurses, other hospital personnel, and visitors wash their hands and instruments, such as stethoscopes, before and after contact with you. Don't feel you are insulting staff and visitors by offering reminders.

You can simply say or post a little sign indicating that your doctors and nurses have instructed you to remind everyone to thoroughly wash their hands for "the safety of all." Hand washing needs to be vigorous, lasting at least fifteen seconds with soap and warm water or with an alcohol sanitizing gel. Antibacterial gel is unnecessary because it is not more effective than soap and may lead to bacteria strains resistant to antibiotics.

Other safeguards to reduce risk of infection include:

a. Keeping a supply of alcohol sanitizing gel near your bedside and encourage everyone to use it.

b. Wash your hands especially well before going to bed and after visits to the bathroom during the night.

c. If you have a surgical wound or an intravenous site, avoid touching it.

d. Make sure your wound dressing, drainage tubes, and catheter sites are dry. Tell your nurse if they become loose or wet.

e. Catheters for supplying nutrients, intravenous medication, and drawing blood should be antiseptic coated. You can ask the nurses about this.

f. Discourage visits from anyone with a head cold or other infection. If your immune system is compromised, visitors may have to wear a mask, hospital gown, and shoe covering.

g. If you have a surgical wound, ask the doctors: "How does my wound look today?" Don't believe the common misperception that "The best way to hide something from a hospital doctor is to put it under a bandage." If necessary, remind your doctor to remove the bandage so the wound can be inspected.

h. Avoid touching the toilet lever, toilet seat, and faucet handles unless you, your advocate, or staff member disinfects them first with alcohol gel.

i. Don't touch the TV remote control or your cell phone unless you wear sterile gloves because they are among the most germ-laden objects in the hospital.

j. Hospital sheets and pillowcases should be changed daily.

Avoiding Medication Errors and Other Errors

Be inquisitive and hypervigilant so you, the most important member of your health care team, can avoid medication and other errors that are common in hospital settings. Enlist the assistance of your health care advocate.

For example, your hospital wristband has bar codes that should correspond with codes of all medications given to you (whether orally, by injection, or by spray). Before being given a drug, politely ask the nurse to double-check your wristband to make sure you are the right patient. Also, periodically ask your nurse or doctor for a copy of your most current medication administration record so you know the names, dosages, and frequencies of your medications. When the nurse gives you a medication, make certain it's on your medication sheet. Don't allow concern about being perceived as mistrustful when in fact you are just making certain that you are being given the correct medication. This will help you (and the staff) avoid unfortunate mistakes.

Also, make certain that any drug allergies you have are noted on your wristband. Before being moved to other sites in the hospital for any tests or procedures, tell your nurse or transporter your full name and last four digits of your social security number. Ask where and for what reason you are being moved.

Because more hospital errors occur during the nursing change of shift, it is especially important to be hypervigilant at those times because important information about you may not be completely and accurately transmitted from one nurse to the other. It bears repeating that hospitals hire locum tenens (temporary) nurses and sometimes physicians (from nearby or distant places) who are less familiar with the procedures and safety measures of the hospital.

Ask the nurse who is winding up his or her shift if there is anything important about your care that you should tell the nurse who is taking over your care. If your principal physician in the hospital is not your usual pcp (who most thoroughly knows you) but rather a hospitalist working under contract at the hospital for a few months or less, you and your advocate should try to be as knowledgeable as possible about your current medical status. If your hospitalist is winding up his or her contracted time at the hospital, encourage him or her to communicate to the "new" hospitalist all the information about your medical status.

Additional Safeguards

After surgery or other procedures that have kept you in bed for days, move out of bed as soon as your physician advises in order to decrease the risk of blood clots in your legs, pulmonary emboli, pneumonia, bedsores, and other complications.

If You Have a Justifiable Complaint

Diplomacy is the better part of valor. Most complaints stem from misunderstandings or miscommunications and can be simply resolved directly with the particular staff member before taking up the issue with someone at a higher level, such as the head nurse or your doctor. It would be reasonable to complain if the nurse doesn't respond within a reasonable time if your intravenous line, which provides you with fluids and medication, becomes infiltrated, causing swelling and discomfort in your arm. Another cause for complaint would be staff members not mindful of washing their hands and not using other hygienic precautions.

If your complaint is not tended to at these levels, and only if you are in a JCAHO-accredited hospital, you can call (anonymously if you prefer) the Joint Commission telephone line weekdays at 800-994-6610 or send an e-mail to complaint@jcaho.org with all the details. Note that the Joint Commission cannot help you if you have a billing or insurance dispute or an interpersonal complaint about a particular staff member.

Billing Questions

Do not be in a rush to pay your bill until you have carefully scrutinized it for errors. Do not be surprised if there is a $10 or higher charge for an aspirin because hospitals have to figure all the costs associated with the order, such as pharmacy, nursing, and administration costs.

If you have medical insurance such as Medicare plus a secondary insurance such as United Health Care or Blue Cross, or perhaps even a tertiary policy, allow sufficient time for the hospital to collect the maximum from these companies before you pay the portion you are responsible for. Some hospital billing departments are more efficient than others, and you want them to be as assertive as possible before you pay the remaining portion. If you pay before the billing department has collected the maximum amounts that the insurance companies are responsible for, the hospital billers may not pursue the insurance companies as aggressively.

If you are still recuperating from your illness when you receive the bills, it may be better to carefully review them (with the assistance of your advocate) once you have fully recovered and feel stronger. Some hospital bills are so difficult to understand that you may need to meet with a knowledgeable official in the hospital's billing department and/or enlist the help of your advocate and accountant. If there is an outstanding balance that is your responsibility, hospitals are more than willing to work out a payment plan rather than lose out on payment or resort to a collection company.

Preparing for a Safe Return Home

Preparing for your return home is equally as important as preparing for your admission to the hospital, and takes even greater planning. Because about 20 percent of hospital patients who have undergone major procedures (such as surgery) suffer a significant complication *after* returning home, be particularly conscientious during this transition.

Pressure from insurance companies and hospitals to control costs has led to shorter and shorter hospital stays. If you or your advocate feels that you are not ready to leave the hospital, you can, in roughly the following order, ask your doctor to extend your stay; ask to talk with someone from the hospital's customer service department; talk with the department's head doctor; or even call your insurance company to explain your reasons.

In the days preceding your return home, think about and write down a list of things you will need to complete before discharge. For example, if you will need to set up a bedroom on the first floor of your home, arrange this beforehand. If you need home visiting services, such as a nurse and/or physical therapist, ask your physician, social worker, or discharge coordinator to arrange this with a home visiting agency, preferably one that is accredited by the JCAHO. Verify that your discharge coordinator, social worker, or your advocate has obtained authorizations for these services from your insurance company.

Before leaving the hospital, ask your doctor who you should contact should you have questions or problems regarding medications, pain, bleeding, or fever; what equipment you will need to take home, such as catheters; and what you may need to arrange for, such as a special bed.

Before discharge, review the discharge plan with both the in-hospital physician (hospitalist) and your personal physician (usually your pcp), who may be primarily responsible for resuming your overall care after your return home. Make certain that you, your family, and your health care advocate all know who will be your principal doctor upon your return home. Request and sign the necessary forms to ensure that your hospital records be faxed or electronically sent immediately to your pcp's office and all physician specialists you see. Transitional periods (such as entering the hospital, change of shift, and especially returning home) are when miscommunication and errors are most likely to occur. When discussing discharge with your doctor, nurse, and social worker, have your health care advocate at your bedside so he or she can take notes and ask questions you may have forgotten. Even consider using a tape recorder so you don't miss important instructions about your post-hospital care.

Of utmost importance is being fully informed about each medication you will be taking (how and when to take it, what side effects to look for, and when the medication can be discontinued). It is crucially important to know whether the medications taken in the hospital should replace the ones you were taking before hospitalization. Don't mistakenly assume that you should resume all the medications you were taking prior to hospitalization. The hospital or pharmacy can provide you with a special plastic medication dispenser, which has compartments for medications to take in the morning, afternoon, and evening. Your nurse may be willing to prepare the dispenser with all the medications to be taken in the coming week. Because many pharmaceutical companies make the same medication but with pills of a different color and shape, be careful not to take double doses of the same medication because they appear different.

The following are examples of additional questions and requests that you (and your advocate) can consider asking your hospital physician before leaving the hospital. This list is not inclusive, and your particular situation may call for additional questions.

1. Do I need to be on a special diet? What about the use of alcohol?

2. When can I resume driving and, if relevant, sexual activity?

3. What complications do I need to be concerned about, what is the likelihood of their occurrence, and what do I need to do about them?

4. When is my follow-up appointment and with whom?

5. If relevant, what special care is required for my operative wound and dressings?

6. If I have an emergency problem, who and what telephone number do I call? Can I contact my doctor at his or her e-mail address?

7. What activities can I resume at home, and when can I return to work?

8. Give the hospital physician a list of all your outpatient physicians, especially your pcp, and all other health professionals who will be working with you following your discharge, and their mailing, fax, e-mail addresses, and telephone numbers. Impress upon your hospital physician (perhaps it was a hospitalist) the extreme importance of sharing all your medical information with

your health professional so your post-hospital care is as coordinated as possible.

Tale of a Successful Hospital Stay

Mrs. Jones, a fifty-year-old obese Chicago housewife married (to a clinical nurse specialist) with three children, had two "gallbladder attacks" before her pcp referred her to a general surgeon, known in the community for being a superb doctor. She and her husband checked out his credentials on the Internet. She obtained confirmation from her insurance company that over 80 percent of all hospital, physician, and other expenses associated with her case were covered.

Since there was no urgency to have gallbladder surgery, she had time to follow through with her surgeon's recommendation to lose thirty-five pounds and to work out at a local gym for overall strengthening, especially of her abdominal muscles. She faithfully avoided foods that would aggravate her gallbladder condition.

Three months later, she selectively informed a few close friends and relatives about her upcoming surgery at a JCAHO-accredited hospital. She left her jewelry and other valuables at home and brought to the hospital a list of all her current medications, health care records, insurance cards, health care directive, and durable power of attorney for health care decisions. She made certain that her pcp shared all her health care information with the surgeon. It was understood by everyone in the hospital that the surgeon and his nurse assistant were responsible for coordinating all aspects of her hospital care and that her husband was her health care advocate.

Mrs. Jones encouraged only a few of her closest friends and relatives to visit, but to refrain from visiting if they had a cold or other infection. Included in her small suitcase was a picture of her family, her cell phone, and several alcohol sanitizers.

She positioned a little sign on her hospital door thanking all for washing their hands. Before taking any medications, she asked the nurse to make certain that the bar code on her wristband matched the code on the medication packet and reminded the nurse of her name and last four digits of her social security number.

She wore sterile gloves when using her cell phone and hospital TV remote control and disinfected the toilet facilities with alcohol gel. When nurses changed shift, she asked the nurse who was leaving what important information should be conveyed to the next nurse on duty.

Her gallbladder surgery was uncomplicated, and she was given permission to walk around her room with assistance from her husband and/or nurse the day after surgery. Her husband took notes when the surgical team reviewed essential information about her transition home. Mrs. Jones and her husband knew what postoperative complications to be mindful of, whom to call, how to care for her abdominal drainage tube and wound, and when she could resume her normal activities. Follow-up appointments were arranged with her surgeon and pcp, who, along with all her other health care professionals, would receive an electronically transmitted discharge summary from the surgeon. It was clear to everyone that her pcp would resume overall coordination of her care after her return home.

PART IV

12

The Value of Getting a Second Opinion

About 30 percent of patients who obtain a second medical opinion discover a diagnosis they didn't know they had. Autopsy studies have shown that 25 percent of patients who die had diseases never diagnosed when they were alive. Yet only 20 percent of patients who obtain medical care each year seek a second opinion.

It has become much easier to obtain a second opinion. Patient records can be quickly sent electronically to another doctor by e-mail or by overnight courier service. It's easier to find experts in various fields of medicine via the Internet. And second opinions are usually relatively inexpensive.

Yet patients don't obtain second opinions for several reasons: fear of acting distrustful of your doctor, concern that he or she will take it as a personal insult, and the need to believe that your doctor is infallible. In addition, you may not realize how worthwhile a second opinion may be or that you are entitled to one. When you are sick, you often feel insure and vulnerable and have a psychological need to over-idealize your physician.

In actuality, a second opinion usually confirms your physician's diagnosis and treatment plan, which increases your confidence in your doctor. When the second opinion differs, it benefits you as well as your primary care physician (pcp), who becomes more knowledgeable about your illness, as the following case illustrates.

Mr. Samuels, a seventy-eight-year-old retired construction worker, visited his elderly long-term physician complaining of pain in his right knee. After examining the knee, his physician said, "You're old; it's expected that you'll have aches and pains." Mr. Samuels replied: "My left knee is seventy-eight years old and doesn't hurt. How do you explain that?" The doctor and patient mutually agreed to get a second opinion from an orthopedic surgeon, who diagnosed and repaired a torn ligament, resulting in the return of the patient's normal, pain-free gait.

In many situations, it is your pcp who is first to recommend obtaining a second opinion, which is often referred to as a "consultation." If a consultation is suggested, there is no reason to feel that your pcp is passing you off to another doctor and does not want to continue in that role. If you're concerned, ask your physician if he or she *will* continue as your primary physician.

Consider getting a second opinion in the following situations: when your illness is not improving, a diagnosis is not forthcoming, communication problems exist between you and your doctor, your doctor is not a specialist in the illness you have, and your intuition and/or your family tells you it's time to seek another opinion.

The following is an example of a second opinion that was lifesaving.

Dr. J, a physician, discovered a small black lesion on his lower leg. He consulted his pcp, who examined the area and reassured Dr. J that there was no cause for concern. No biopsy was performed. A month later, Dr. J sought a second opinion from a dermatologist, who recommended a biopsy. Dr. J was found to have a virulent form of melanoma and had surgery two days later to have it removed. A year later there has not been a recurrence.

Some examples of frequently missed diagnoses include depression, early signs of cognitive impairment, osteoporosis (the initial sign may be a fracture), hypothyroidism (low functioning of the thyroid gland), sexually transmitted diseases, cancer, and type-2 (adult onset) diabetes.

If you have a long-term, trusting relationship with your pcp, include him or her in the process of obtaining a second opinion, especially if you want to continue under your doctor's care. Ask your doctor who he or she would see in consultation for the same medical condition that you have. Your pcp can facilitate the referral and obtain valuable feedback from the consultant that can positively influence your future medical care. However, you want to avoid being the "messenger" between your pcp and the consultant; rather you should encourage their communication. Ask the consultant to write a letter to your pcp with a copy to you. If your pcp has known you for a long time, he or she may be better able than the consultant to communicate to you the consultant's findings in a meaningful and empathic manner that takes into consideration your medical, psychological, sociocultural, and spiritual background.

Try to find a Board-certified physician who specializes in the illness that you have. You can use any number of Internet sites, such as the American Medical Association – www.ama-assn.org; then go to "Patients," then to "Doctor Finder." Other web sites are listed at the end of this chapter.

Before your appointment with a consultant, have your pcp send to the consultant all your pertinent records. To prepare to see the consultant, write down notes that include the history of the onset of your symptoms, the course of the illness, treatments tried, and current medications.

After the consultant reviews all the information and examines you, he or she may order additional tests and discuss your case with your pcp. If you decide that you want the consultant or one of his or her colleagues to take over your care, this needs to be understood by all so the transition can be seamless.

Regarding payment for a second opinion, most insurance plans will cover the cost, but it's wise to read your policy and/or speak with a supervisor at your insurance company. Some insurers actually require you to get a second opinion before paying for very expensive procedures, such as cardiac bypass surgery or a kidney or liver transplant. Many insurance plans won't pay for a second opinion, so you may have to bear the costs. But if your life is at stake, it's worth the investment.

Use the Internet to learn as much as possible about your medical condition. Web sites often provide the most up-to-date research and list the researchers carrying out the latest clinical studies that pertain to your diagnosis and treatment. The most useful and reliable Internet sites for finding the latest information are not sites with the designation ".com", which indicates a commercial site whose motivation is to sell you something. Be wary of companies selling products touted by movie stars or athletes based on hyped-up testimonials claiming 100 percent success rates. The most reliable information is found on Internet sites indicated by ".edu" (indicating an educational institution) or by ".gov" (indicating a U.S. government site) and ".org" sites (which are not-for-profit organizations). Even for sites indicated by ".edu", ".gov", or ".org", you should check to see that the information is current, identifies the source of the information (for example, studies carried out at such acclaimed medical centers as Johns Hopkins or the Mayo Clinic), and that the articles are published in refereed journals.

Regarding clinical studies that pertain to your illness, the most reliable are double-blind, randomized, controlled studies of a large number of patients carried out at respected medical centers. Studies carried out in the United States, in contrast to those overseas, often adhere to stricter research standards.

In addition to the American Medical Association web site, other valuable web sites include:
www.uptodate.com – Up-to-date reference on medical conditions with excellent information from scientific literature. Go to "Benefits for Patients" section.

www.cdc.gov/ncidod/diseases – The Centers for Disease Control provide information about various infectious diseases.

www.drugs.com – Includes drug information for over-the-counter and prescription drugs.

www.cancer.gov– The National Cancer Institute provides information about types of cancer, including treatment, coping, and current clinical research trials.

www.nia.nih.gov – The National Institute on Aging (NIA) provides valuable information on health and diseases associated with aging and how to seek enrollment in clinical trials.

www.psych.org – The American Psychiatric Association (APA) site provides information on psychiatric disorders, district branches where you can obtain referrals, and a myriad of other topics.

www.aagponline.org – The American Association for Geriatric Psychiatry (AAGP) provides a list of psychiatrists who specialize in the psychiatric treatment of the elderly and information about common disorders. Telephone 301-654-7850.

13

Complementary and Alternative Treatment Approaches

T he term *complementary and alternative medicine* – CAM (also referred to as non-traditional, integrative, and holistic medicine)--refers to various treatment approaches whose methods and efficacy differ from those of traditional medicine. Although most claims about the clinical benefits and safety of these non-traditional approaches have not been proven scientifically, some CAM practices are used in conjunction with traditional medical approaches.

Complementary and alternative medicine approaches are being used by an increasing number of people in the United States and other countries. Within the past decade or so, more than one third of Americans used one or more forms of alternative treatment each year, but less than 20 percent informed their regular physician.

Why are patients often reluctant to inform their primary care physician (pcp) about considering an alternative treatment? They might be concerned about offending their physician, or they think that their doctor will frown on their interest in alternative approaches. They "forget" to inform their physician because they think it's not important to do so.

But it *is* extremely important to inform your regular doctor(s) before using a non-traditional approach because some treatments, such as herbs and over-the-counter medicines, may have detrimental interactions with prescription medicines. In addition, traditional physicians have become more knowledgeable about the potential value and risks of CAMs, and may make referrals to, and work collaboratively with, reputable practitioners in the community. Discussing your interest with your pcp facilitates coordination of your health care. Also, some insurance companies require a referral from your physician in order for the non-traditional treatment to be covered.

CAMs have become increasingly popular in the United States for several reasons. Some approaches have been scientifically proven to be effective; many of them have been used for centuries; non-traditional practitioners may spend more time and listen more attentively to patients than do busy pcp's; faith and hope may be major factors that contribute to the success of these treatments (some call it the placebo effect); and some treatments may be particularly helpful for patients with chronic problems, such as low back pain.

The widespread use of CAMs led the United States to establish the National Center for Complementary and Alternative Medicine (NCCAM) within the National Institutes of Health (NIH) to evaluate the effectiveness and safety of these non-traditional healing practices, to understand scientifically the reasons for their effectiveness, and to inform the public about their findings. A NCCAM study found the most prominent forms of CAM used in the United States were praying for one's own health or the health of others (more than 60 percent of those using a CAM approach), using natural products (such as echinacea, ginseng, *Gingko biloba* (19 percent), deep breathing exercises (12 percent), meditation (8 percent), and chiropractic treatment (8 percent). Many Americans use two or more approaches. The study also found the most common conditions treated were back, head, and neck pain. Most users of CAM believed that the greatest benefits were achieved when CAM was combined with conventional medical treatment.

Additional NCCAM studies have validated that acupuncture is beneficial to those with functional impairment and osteoarthritic pain of the knee; combined glucosamine and chondroitin sulfate benefits a small group of patients with more severe osteoarthritic pain; and St.-John's-wort is not effective for major depression (although it may be effective for mild depression).

Unfortunately, the vast majority of CAMs are not based on scientific studies, and some are considered quackery. Without scientific evidence, many physicians view many of these non-traditional methods with some skepticism. On the other hand, more than half of U.S. traditional medical schools provide some education about alternative medicine, and some are carrying out research to determine which approaches have scientific merit.

Some health maintenance organizations (HMOs) have approved alternative treatments for reimbursement, such as acupuncture and chiropractic treatment and allow patients to visit alternative practitioners without needing a referral by their pcp. Check this out with your insurance company.

The more commonly used CAM approaches discussed in this chapter include chiropractics, acupuncture, naturopathy, homeopathy, massage, meditation, prayer, and the use of special diets, herbs, and vitamins.

Finding an Alternative Practitioner

Ask for recommendations from your pcp, family, and friends familiar with the medical community. Just like selecting your pcp, you want to know how long your prospective practitioner has been in practice and if he or she is licensed in your state. You can call your state's licensing and professional regulation office to ascertain if the practitioner is properly licensed. Use the Internet to check the practitioner's education and experience. Ask if the alternative practitioner is willing to work collaboratively with your pcp. If you don't get satisfactory answers to your inquiries, consider finding someone else.

Learn about the benefits and risks of the alternative therapy before arranging a first appointment by contacting NCCAM's Internet site (www.nccam.nih.gov). Then go to "Health Information," then "Safe Use of Complementary Health Products and Practices."

In the final analysis, after much thought and investigation, you need to decide if a CAM can be worthwhile for you. The following is a summary of some of the more common CAM approaches.

Chiropractic

Chiropractic is concerned with the diagnosis, treatment, and prevention of disorders of the musculoskeletal system, especially disorders of the spine and the effects of these disorders on general health. Chiropractors diagnose illness by X-rays and clinical examination. Treatment involves manual manipulation of the spine, bones, musculature, and joints to restore biomechanical function.

Chiropractic is the largest alternative health profession in the United States, with over 50,000 practitioners. Four or five years of study at one of about sixteen accredited chiropractic colleges is required, followed by passing a four-part exam. Chiropractors need to be licensed in the state where they practice. Some states and insurance policies give chiropractors more leeway (to be a pcp and to receive insurance payments) than others. Some research suggests that chiropractors are just as effective as traditional physicians at helping back pain sufferers. A good source of information about chiropractors is the Federation of Chiropractic Licensing Boards (www.fclb.org).

Acupuncture

Acupuncture is a Chinese healing technique dating back to 5000 BC and continues to be an important medical intervention in the eastern part of the world and also one of the most popular and regulated CAMs in the United States. Acupuncturists insert sterilized silver or gold needles, some as thin as a human hair, into the skin at varying depths and rotate them or leave them in place for varying periods of time.

It is believed that the needles stimulate the release of endorphins and enkephalins to relieve pain and to alleviate symptoms of some illnesses. The benefits have been validated for pain management, fibromyalgia, headache, osteoarthritis of the knee, and postoperative nausea and vomiting. Most pain management clinics in England and many in the United States use acupuncture in their arsenal of approaches. Acupuncture is also used for smoking cessation and relieving the symptoms of substance abuse, as well as insomnia, anxiety, depression, and asthma. Thousands of physicians in the United States have taken special training courses and include acupuncture as part of their practice.

To become licensed, about sixteen states require a degree from a school for acupuncture and Oriental medicine accredited by the Accreditation Commission for Acupuncture and Oriental Medicine (ACAOM). Graduates do not have a medical degree. They practice other modes of Oriental medicine, including herbal remedies. To find out what your state requires for licensing and other information, check the National Certification Commission for Acupuncture and Oriental Medicine (NCCAOM) at www.nccaom.org.

Some states require your pcp to refer you to an acupuncturist before your insurance will consider paying for it, so check with your insurer. As with other CAMs, discuss your interest with your physician before considering treatment.

My friend's ninety-four-year-old mother suffered a fracture of her lower spine ten years ago. Surgery was recommended by a busy, authoritative orthopedic surgeon who became impatient when she questioned the need for surgery and refused to sign the consent form. She has been symptom free using acupuncture treatments four times a year up to the present.

Naturopathy

Naturopathy is based on the belief that the body has the power to heal itself. Naturopaths advocate some combination of healthy nutrition, pollution-free air and water, regular exercise, hot/cold compresses, colonic irrigation (such as enemas), massage therapy, herbs, and rest therapy.

There are only a few naturopathic colleges in the United States that are accredited by the Council on Naturopathic Medical Education (CNME). Four years of postgraduate training is required followed by passing an examination.

As of 2008, only sixteen U.S. states, the District of Columbia, and Puerto Rico have laws that license graduates of American naturopathic medical schools to practice. You can find out your state's status at the American Association of Naturopathic Physicians (AANP) -- www.naturopathic.org.

Because no standard regulations of the field exist, persons with minimal or no special training can set up a practice in some states and call themselves doctors. Many traditionally trained physicians think it is confusing to the public when naturopathic practitioners call themselves doctors because they don't have the same rigorous training, education, and licensing requirements.

Homeopathy

Homeopathy is based on the concept that self-healing is a basic characteristic of human life. Extremely small doses of special medicines are used, many derived from plants (such as ergot fungus) and minerals (such as silver and iodine) that help the body build defenses against particular diseases. Medications are prepared as tinctures (that is, mixed with 95 percent grain alcohol) or as pills. Research has shown that such highly diluted substances may have no greater benefit than a placebo. However, homeopathic medications are used throughout the world and are prescribed by other alternative practitioners. Many patients claim that these medications are very effective.

I know a physician in Maine who pooh-poohed homeopathy for years until he became so uncomfortable with a medical condition that traditional medicine could not address that he gave in to a friend's urging and tried homeopathy. It worked so well that he now practices homeopathy as well as traditional medicine.

Only a few states offer licensing for homeopaths, but there are over 6,000 in the United States. Most are practitioners in another field, such as chiropractic, who incorporate some aspects of homeopathy into their work.

Homeopathic medicines are sold over-the-counter in the United States and in other parts of the world. As with other CAM treatments, talk with your pcp before using homeopathic medications to make certain they don't interfere with your other medications. And keep your physician informed to ensure overall coordination of your medical care.

Massage Therapy

Some believe that massage therapy affects the body by increasing circulation and lymphatic flow, improving the tone of the musculoskeletal system, and producing a tranquilizing effect on the mind. There are many different types, such as Swedish, Oriental, Shiatsu, and Esalen, but they are more similar than different. Some studies have shown that massage therapy can reduce anxiety and pain perception.

Most people find massage physically and mentally rejuvenating, but it does not cure any medical illness. Credentialing requirements vary widely in the United States. About half the states require classroom education, supervised training at an institution accredited by the Commission on Massage Therapy Accreditation (COMTA), and an examination, but half the states have no credentialing requirements. To check on your state's status, contact the National Certification Board for Therapeutic Massage and Bodywork---NCBTMB---www.ncbtmb.com.

Meditation

Meditation is a technique that lets you enter a trance-like state by focusing on a word, sound, object, or your natural breathing. Upon entering this state, you experience calm, reduced anxiety, and sometimes reduced blood pressure and respiratory rate.

Some people practice meditation daily and report that it reduces stress-related disorders. Small and large workshops are given all over the United States. Personally, I have found it a pleasant and simple way of reducing tension and anxiety, especially after stressful days.

Prayer

For centuries, prayer and visits to religious shrines to find relief from suffering and pain support the widespread belief that spirituality helps the healing process.

Some advocate the use of silent, shared, and distant prayer (praying on behalf of someone else for a specific purpose) to benefit those who are sick and suffering. A study of inner city homeless women found that 48 percent reported that prayer significantly reduced depression and their use of alcohol and drugs.

Twelve-step programs for those with alcohol and/or drug addictions have a long history of using prayer and spirituality as an important component. Studies have shown that personal religious beliefs and regular attendance at places of worship contribute to a decreased incidence of high blood pressure and depression.

Persons with a lifetime of practicing their strong religious beliefs, contrasted with lifelong non-believers, will obviously find it more beneficial to turn to their spiritual convictions during times of sickness and stress.

Diet and Nutrition

Dietary supplements are products that contain vitamins, minerals, and amino acids that are intended to supplement, rather than substitute for, a healthy diet or a balanced meal. Multivitamins are often components of a vast array of other compounds that can be purchased from grocery and health food stores, pharmacies, and on the Internet. About 75 percent of Americans use some form of nutritional supplements. The medical benefits of these products vary greatly in their safety and efficacy.

Special diets have an important place in modern medicine. Alternative diets, some with specific vitamin and mineral supplements, have been developed to help patients with specific diseases. Diets low in fat are recommended for the treatment of diabetes and vascular and heart disease. The Pritikin diet is very low in fat and high in fiber and complex carbohydrates. The Atkins diet is low in carbohydrates and high in protein and has proven to be effective in short-term weight loss, but it lacks long-term studies on its effect on health. All these diets have their advocates, and their popularity changes over time. Studies have shown that weight loss alone can decrease blood pressure and cholesterol and sometimes reduce (and sometimes eliminate) the need for drugs in newly diagnosed adult-onset diabetes.

Scientific studies have substantiated the efficacy of some special diets. Those following a strictly vegetarian diet may be deficient in certain vitamins and proteins, so supplementing the diet with vitamin B12 and essential amino acids is suggested. Americans leading a busy lifestyle have been shown to be missing the minimum required amount of some vitamins and minerals. Some nutritional experts recommend taking a high-quality multivitamin with minerals once or twice daily. Some advocate taking it twice daily because several vitamins dissolve in water and are excreted by the kidneys within twelve hours.

With the exception of some basic vitamins (A, C, D, E, B1, B5, B6, B12, folate, and niacin) and some minerals (iron, potassium, magnesium, calcium, and selenium), there is limited information about the value of most vitamin and mineral supplements on the market. When choosing a multivitamin and mineral for daily use, consider one that has most of the above ingredients.

Fortunately, for many vitamins, minerals, and other nutrients, the federal government has established recommended daily allowances (RDAs) necessary to meet the nutritional needs for the average middle-aged U.S. citizen. For the majority of Americans, a diet rich in whole grains, lean meat, fish, and green vegetables is recommended. Discouraged is an excess intake of fatty foods and sugar products (plentiful in breakfast cereals, cookies, and soft drinks).

Vitamin Deficiencies

Vitamin deficiencies often affect the malnourished and alcohol and drug abusers. For example, alcoholics are often deficient in Vitamin B1 (thiamine), contributing to delirium, sometimes brain damage, and even beriberi. If diagnosed early, these conditions can be improved with thiamine pills, abstinence, and improved diet. Deficiency of vitamin B12 or folic acid can cause depression, anemia, and delirium that can progress to dementia if not diagnosed early and treated. Deficiency of vitamin D and calcium can cause osteoporosis and bone fracture, especially in post-menopausal women. Exercise, supplemental vitamin D, and special medications can help reduce the risk.

Precautions about Dietary Supplements

In contrast to prescription drugs, which are subjected to rigorous scientific studies and years of scrutiny by the Food and Drug Administration (FDA) before approval to be marketed, manufacturers of nutritional products can simply package and sell their product. Since 1994 the Dietary Supplemental Health and Education Act (DSHEA) has permitted herbal and other such remedies to be sold in the United States as "food products." The FDA has little to no authority or budget to monitor these nutritional supplements.

Fortunately, one precaution you can take when buying a nutritional supplement is to look for the label on the container that indicates the product is "USP-verified." This signifies that a nonprofit organization, the U.S. Pharmacopeia, has confirmed that the pill contains what the manufacturer claims it has, although it doesn't make a judgment as to whether or not it's effective. Taking large doses of vitamins can have negative consequences, so using them in moderation is preferable and safer.

Consider getting your doctor's opinion about trying a special diet, nutritional supplement, or one or more of the thousands of herbal products on the market. One reason is that some herbal remedies can interfere with the actions of your prescribed medications.

For example, some dietary supplements and herbal remedies can increase the risk of bleeding during and after surgery, so surgeons often recommend stopping these at least a week before and a period of time after surgery. Substances that can increase the risk of bleeding include glucosamine, ginseng, *Ginkgo biloba*, ginger, and garlic, as well as vitamin E, DHEA, EPA, and St.-John's-wort. The latter, sometimes used for mild depression, can interfere with the action of warfarin (a blood thinner), diminish the effectiveness of birth control pills, and cause serious side effects (including hypertension) if used with prescribed antidepressants.

Since many herbal remedies find their way into breast milk, physicians often advise pregnant and breast-feeding women to avoid herbal medicines during pregnancy and lactation. Discuss this precaution with your doctor.

For the majority of dietary supplements and herbal remedies, whether or not they work is part conjecture and part faith. A woman friend of mine suffered a brain injury years ago and greatly benefited from years of meditation. She continues to spend $600 of her $2,000 monthly income on dietary supplements and herbal remedies and is absolutely convinced that she couldn't bear reducing or going without them. Faith and hope probably play a significant role in her continued recovery.

To find out the benefits and risks of vitamins, dietary supplements, and special diets, enter the specific supplement into your Internet browser, and look for sites ending in ".edu" or ".gov." These suffixes indicate an education or U.S. government site, respectively, which are more credible than ".com" sites, which are commercial sites wanting to sell you something. As with other CAMs, it's worthwhile to first discuss your options with your physician.

14

The Future of Health Care in America

O ne provision of the Affordable Care Act (ACA) mandates that almost all Americans will have health insurance by the year 2014. Because there will be a shortage of primary care physicians (pcp's) to serve this increased patient population, clinical nurse specialists, physician assistants, and other health professionals will have an expanded role, such as providing initial medical and psychiatric evaluations and treating less serious medical problems before patients are evaluated by the pcp.

Even if innovative models of health care delivery, discussed in Chapter 1, result in better patient outcomes, it may take years until these treatment approaches become the new standard of care for Medicare and other insurance plans. Medicare can then use its market presence and governmental support to promulgate these programs to private and state-supported insurance companies.

Big business, in the form of large hospital corporations and pharmaceutical and insurance companies, will continue to play a dominate role in how health care is provided. They have the financial means to support the election campaigns of congressional candidates who advocate legislation favorable to their companies.

The role of the solo practitioner in private practice will continue to diminish and be replaced by large health care organizations such as the Mayo Clinic and the Kaiser Foundation. Big hospital corporations will continue to buy out the practices of solo practitioners and physician groups. These physicians then become employees of the hospital corporations. Solo practitioners and physician groups are enticed to become hospital employees because of guaranteed salaries, reduced administrative paperwork, vacations, insurance, retirement, and other benefits. Having control of physicians in a community will ensure more patient referrals to the hospitals that pay the physicians' salaries.

More and more large corporations, looking for ways to reduce absenteeism from work and reduce health care costs of its employees, are rewarding workers who participate in health-promoting programs, such as weight reduction and alcohol, drug, and smoking cessation programs. Employees who are successful in these and other preventative programs and agree to practice a healthier lifestyle will be financially rewarded by paying lower health insurance premiums and, ideally, living longer, healthier, more productive lives. According to the Kaiser Family Foundation, nearly 90 percent of large companies now offer wellness programs.

Medical and hospital practices will be more computerized, which directly benefits patients by reducing errors and disseminating patient information more quickly and efficiently. The U.S. Department of Health and Human Services has been working on a national health information network that will allow consenting Americans to have all their past and current medical information accessible on the Internet. When this is eventually put into place, were you to transfer your health care to a new physician and give permission, your new doctor would have immediate access to all your health care records. Currently, you can store all your health care information on a Smartphone, computer chip, or credit-card-size card.

Safeguards will need to be put in place to ensure confidentiality.

Given these and other changes in health care delivery, what can you, your family, and I do to take advantage of these hoped-for improvements? First and foremost is having a pcp who cares about you and is invested in keeping you and your family healthy. Your physician should spend adequate time with you and listen to your concerns. Your physician and his or her staff should be dependable, inform you of test results, give you follow-up appointments, and coordinate your care with other health professionals.

Whether or not health insurance is provided to you and your family by your employer or you purchase it on your own, obtain the most comprehensive insurance you can afford. Keep in mind that ever-increasing medical expenses are the number one cause of bankruptcy in America.

Selecting the best affordable health insurance can be bewildering, so consider enlisting the services of a trusted, independent insurance agent to help you make the best decisions, or talk with a knowledgeable person in your company's human resources department.

Become and stay healthy by eating nutritional foods, exercising regularly, having goals in life you feel passionate about, and diligently complying with your physician's recommendations. Scientific discoveries about how to have a healthier, happier lifestyle have contributed to the increased longevity of each successive generation. For example, my grandparents--immigrants from Eastern Europe in the late 1800s--knew nothing about exercise, diet, and the dangers of smoking. My father was an athlete throughout high school and college, but he didn't continue regular exercise once he entered professional life. He didn't give up smoking until age sixty. I need to push myself to exercise regularly. My three adult children are in excellent physical health, exercise daily, eat nutritional foods, and don't smoke or drink.

We all need to overcome denying our vulnerability to misfortune and accept our mortality. We need to stop rationalizing our unhealthy choices, and adopt a healthier lifestyle for ourselves and our families to make us all more resilient to illness. I hope the information shared with you in this book will enable you and your family to live healthier, happier, and more productive lives.

Appendix I

OPTIONAL ADVANCE HEALTH-CARE DIRECTIVE

Explanation

You have the right to give instructions about your own health care. You also have the right to name someone else to make health-care decisions for you. This form lets you do either or both of these things. It also lets you express your wishes regarding the designation of your primary physician.

THIS FORM IS OPTIONAL. Each paragraph and word of this form is also optional. If you use this form, you may cross out, complete or modify all or any part of it. You are free to use a different form. If you use this form, be sure to sign it and date it.

PART 1 of this form is a power of attorney for health care. PART 1 lets you name another individual as agent to make health-care decisions for you if you become incapable of making your own decisions or if you want someone else to make those decisions for you now even though you are still capable. You may also name an alternate agent to act for you if your first choice is not willing, able or reasonably available to make decisions for you. Unless related to you, your agent may not be an owner, operator or employee of a health-care institution at which you are receiving care.

Unless the form you sign limits the authority of your agent, your agent may make all health-care decisions for you. This form has a place for you to limit the authority of your agent. You need not limit the authority of your agent if you wish to rely on your agent for all health-care decisions that may have to be made. If you choose not to limit the authority of your agent, your agent will have the right to:

(a)   consent or refuse consent to any care, treatment, service or procedure to maintain, diagnose or otherwise affect a physical or mental condition;

(b)   select or discharge health-care providers and institutions;

(c)   approve or disapprove diagnostic tests, surgical procedures, programs of medication and orders not to resuscitate; and

(d)   direct the provision, withholding or withdrawal of artificial nutrition and hydration and all other forms of health care.

THIS FORM IS OPTIONAL. You do not have to use any form; instead, you may tell your doctor who you want to make health care decisions for you. If you have not signed a form or told your doctor who you want to make your health care decisions, New Mexico law allows these people, in the following order, to make your health care decisions (if these people are reasonably available): 1) spouse, 2) significant others, 3) adult child, 4) parent, 5) adult brother or sister, 6) grandparent, 7) close friend.

PART 2 of this form lets you give specific instructions about any aspect of your health care. Choices are provided for you to express your wishes regarding life-sustaining treatment, including the provision of artificial nutrition and hydration, as well as the provision of pain relief. In addition, you may express your wishes regarding whether you want to make an anatomical gift of some or all of your organs and tissue. Space is also provided for you to add to the choices you have made or for you to write out any additional wishes.

PART 3 of this form lets you designate a physician to have primary responsibility for your health care.

After completing this form, sign and date the form at the end. It is recommended but not required that you request two other individuals to sign as witnesses. Give a copy of the signed and completed form to your physician, to any other health-care providers you may have, to any health-care institution at which you are receiving care and to any health-care agents you have named. You should talk to the person you have named as agent to make sure that he or she understands your wishes and is willing to take the responsibility.

You have the right to revoke this advance health-care directive or replace this form at any time.

* *

PART 1

POWER OF ATTORNEY FOR HEALTH CARE

(1)   DESIGNATION OF AGENT: I designate the following individual as my agent to make health-care decisions for me:

_____

(name of individual you choose as agent)

_____

(address)   (city)   (state)   (zip code)

_____

(home phone)   (work phone)

If I revoke my agent's authority or if my agent is not willing, able or reasonably available to make a health-care decision for me, I designate as my first alternate agent:

_____

(name of individual you choose as first alternate agent)

_____

(address)   (city)   (state)   (zip code)

_____

(home phone)   (work phone)

If I revoke the authority of my agent and first alternate agent or if neither is willing, able or reasonably available to make a health-care decision for me, I designate as my second alternate agent:

_____

(name of individual you choose as second alternate agent)

_____

(address)   (city)   (state)   (zip code)

_____

(home phone)   (work phone)

(2)   AGENT'S AUTHORITY: My agent is authorized to obtain and review medical records, reports and information about me and to make all health-care decisions for me, including decisions to provide, withhold or withdraw artificial nutrition, hydration and all other forms of health care to keep me alive, except as I state here:

_____

_____

(Add additional sheets if needed.)

(3)   WHEN AGENT'S AUTHORITY BECOMES EFFECTIVE: My agent's authority becomes effective when my primary physician and one other qualified health-care professional determine that I am unable to make my own health-care decisions. If I initial this box [ ], my agent's authority to make health-care decisions for me takes effect immediately.

(4)   AGENT'S OBLIGATION: My agent shall make health-care decisions for me in accordance with this power of attorney for health care, any instructions I give in Part 2 of this form and my other wishes to the extent known to my agent. To the extent my wishes are unknown, my agent shall make health-care decisions for me in accordance with what my agent determines to be in my best interest. In determining my best interest, my agent shall consider my personal values to the extent known to my agent.

(5)   NOMINATION OF GUARDIAN: If a guardian of my person needs to be appointed for me by a court, I nominate the agent designated in this form. If that agent is not willing, able or reasonably available to act as guardian, I nominate the alternate agents whom I have named, in the order designated.

PART 2

INSTRUCTIONS FOR HEALTH CARE

If you are satisfied to allow your agent to determine what is best for you in making end-of-life decisions, you need not fill out this part of the form. If you do fill out this part of the form, you may cross out any wording you do not want.

(6)   END-OF-LIFE DECISIONS: If I am unable to make or communicate decisions regarding my health care, and IF (i) I have an incurable or irreversible condition that will result in my death within a relatively short time, OR (ii) I become unconscious and, to a reasonable degree of medical certainty, I will not regain consciousness, OR (iii) the likely risks and burdens of treatment would outweigh the expected benefits, THEN I direct that my health-care providers and others involved in my care provide, withhold or withdraw treatment in accordance with the choice I have initialed below in one of the following three boxes:

    [ ]   I CHOOSE NOT To Prolong Life
       I do not want my life to be prolonged.
    [ ]   I CHOOSE To Prolong Life
       I want my life to be prolonged as long as possible within the limits of generally accepted health-care standards.
    [ ]   I CHOOSE To Let My Agent Decide
       My agent under my power of attorney for health care may make life-sustaining treatment decisions for me.

(7)   ARTIFICIAL NUTRITION AND HYDRATION: If I have chosen above NOT to prolong life, I also specify by marking my initials below:

    [ ]   I DO NOT want artificial nutrition OR
    [ ]   I DO want artificial nutrition.
    [ ]   I DO NOT want artificial hydration unless required for my comfort OR
    [ ]   I DO want artificial hydration.

(8)   RELIEF FROM PAIN: Regardless of the choices I have made in this form and except as I state in the following space, I direct that the best medical care possible to keep me clean, comfortable and free of pain or discomfort be provided at all times so that my dignity is maintained, even if this care hastens my death:

_____

_____

(9)   ANATOMICAL GIFT DESIGNATION: Upon my death I specify as marked below whether I choose to make an anatomical gift of all or some of my organs or tissue:

[ ]   I CHOOSE to make an anatomical gift of all of my organs or tissue to be determined by medical suitability at the time of death, and artificial support may be maintained long enough for organs to be removed.

[ ]   I CHOOSE to make a partial anatomical gift of some of my organs and tissue as specified below, and artificial support may be maintained long enough for organs to be removed.

_____

_____

[ ]   I REFUSE to make an anatomical gift of any of my organs or tissue.
[ ]   I CHOOSE to let my agent decide.

(10)   OTHER WISHES: (If you wish to write your own instructions, or if you wish to add to the instructions you have given above, you may do so here.) I direct that:

_____

_____

(Add additional sheets if needed.)

PART 3

PRIMARY PHYSICIAN

(11)   I designate the following physician as my primary physician:

_____

(name of physician)

_____

(address)   (city)   (state)   (zip code)

_____

(phone)

If the physician I have designated above is not willing, able or reasonably available to act as my primary physician, I designate the following physician as my primary physician:

_____

(name of physician)

_____

(address)   (city)   (state)   (zip code)

_____

(phone)

* *

(12)   EFFECT OF COPY: A copy of this form has the same effect as the original.

(13)   REVOCATION: I understand that I may revoke this OPTIONAL ADVANCE HEALTH-CARE DIRECTIVE at any time, and that if I revoke it, I should promptly notify my supervising health-care provider and any health-care institution where I am receiving care and any others to whom I have given copies of this power of attorney. I understand that I may revoke the designation of an agent either by a signed writing or by personally informing the supervising health-care provider.

(14)   SIGNATURES: Sign and date the form here:

_____   _____

(date)   (sign your name)

_____   _____

(address)   (print your name)

_____   _____

(city)   (state)   (your social security number)

(Optional) SIGNATURES OF WITNESSES:

First witness   Second witness

_____   _____

(print your name)   (print your name)

_____   _____

(address)   (address)

_____   _____

(city)   (state)   (city)   (state)

_____   _____

(signature of witness)   (signature of witness)

_____   _____

(date)   (date)".

Appendix II

POLST (Physician Orders for Life-Sustaining Treatment) and directions for completing the form (HIPAA Permits Disclosure Form)

HIPAA PERMITS DISCLOSURE OF POLST TO OTHER HEALTH CARE PROVIDERS AS NECESSARY

Physician Orders for Life-Sustaining Treatment (POLST)

EMSA #111 B
(Effective 4/1/2011)

First follow these orders, then contact physician. This is a Physician Order Sheet based on the person's current medical condition and wishes. Any section not completed implies full treatment for that section. A copy of the signed POLST form is legal and valid. POLST complements an Advance Directive and is not intended to replace that document. Everyone shall be treated with dignity and respect.

Patient Last Name:	Date Form Prepared:
Patient First Name:	Patient Date of Birth:
Patient Middle Name:	Medical Record #: *(optional)*

A
Check One

CARDIOPULMONARY RESUSCITATION (CPR): *If person has no pulse and is not breathing.*
When NOT in cardiopulmonary arrest, follow orders in Sections B and C.
☐ **Attempt Resuscitation/CPR** (Selecting CPR in Section A **requires** selecting Full Treatment in Section B)
☐ **Do Not Attempt Resuscitation/DNR** (Allow Natural Death)

B
Check One

MEDICAL INTERVENTIONS: *If person has pulse and/or is breathing.*
☐ **Comfort Measures Only** Relieve pain and suffering through the use of medication by any route, positioning, wound care and other measures. Use oxygen, suction and manual treatment of airway obstruction as needed for comfort. *Transfer to hospital only if comfort needs cannot be met in current location.*
☐ **Limited Additional Interventions** In addition to care described in Comfort Measures Only, use medical treatment, antibiotics, and IV fluids as indicated. Do not intubate. May use non-invasive positive airway pressure. Generally avoid intensive care.
  ☐ *Transfer to hospital only if comfort needs cannot be met in current location.*
☐ **Full Treatment** In addition to care described in Comfort Measures Only and Limited Additional Interventions, use intubation, advanced airway interventions, mechanical ventilation, and defibrillation/cardioversion as indicated. *Transfer to hospital if indicated. Includes intensive care.*

Additional Orders: _____

C
Check One

ARTIFICIALLY ADMINISTERED NUTRITION: *Offer food by mouth if feasible and desired.*
☐ No artificial means of nutrition, including feeding tubes. Additional Orders:_____
☐ Trial period of artificial nutrition, including feeding tubes. _____
☐ Long-term artificial nutrition, including feeding tubes. _____

D

INFORMATION AND SIGNATURES:

Discussed with: ☐ Patient (Patient Has Capacity)   ☐ Legally Recognized Decisionmaker

☐ Advance Directive dated _____ available and reviewed →   Health Care Agent if named in Advance Directive:
☐ Advance Directive not available   Name: _____
☐ No Advance Directive   Phone: _____

Signature of Physician
My signature below indicates to the best of my knowledge that these orders are consistent with the person's medical condition and preferences.

Print Physician Name:	Physician Phone Number:	Physician License Number:
Physician Signature: *(required)*		Date:

Signature of Patient or Legally Recognized Decisionmaker
By signing this form, the legally recognized decisionmaker acknowledges that this request regarding resuscitative measures is consistent with the known desires of, and with the best interest of, the individual who is the subject of the form.

Print Name:		Relationship: *(write self if patient)*
Signature: *(required)*		Date:
Address:	Daytime Phone Number:	Evening Phone Number:

SEND FORM WITH PERSON WHENEVER TRANSFERRED OR DISCHARGED

HIPAA PERMITS DISCLOSURE OF POLST TO OTHER HEALTH CARE PROVIDERS AS NECESSARY

Patient Information

Name (last, first, middle):	Date of Birth:	Gender: M F

Health Care Provider Assisting with Form Preparation

Name:	Title:	Phone Number:

Additional Contact

Name:	Relationship to Patient:	Phone Number:

Directions for Health Care Provider

Completing POLST

- Completing a POLST form is voluntary. California law requires that a POLST form be followed by health care providers, and provides immunity to those who comply in good faith. In the hospital setting, a patient will be assessed by a physician who will issue appropriate orders.
- POLST does not replace the Advance Directive. When available, review the Advance Directive and POLST form to ensure consistency, and update forms appropriately to resolve any conflicts.
- POLST must be completed by a health care provider based on patient preferences and medical indications.
- A legally recognized decisionmaker may include a court-appointed conservator or guardian, agent designated in an Advance Directive, orally designated surrogate, spouse, registered domestic partner, parent of a minor, closest available relative, or person whom the patient's physician believes best knows what is in the patient's best interest and will make decisions in accordance with the patient's expressed wishes and values to the extent known.
- POLST must be signed by a physician and the patient or decisionmaker to be valid. Verbal orders are acceptable with follow-up signature by physician in accordance with facility/community policy.
- Certain medical conditions or treatments may prohibit a person from residing in a residential care facility for the elderly.
- If a translated form is used with patient or decisionmaker, attach it to the signed English POLST form.
- Use of original form is strongly encouraged. Photocopies and FAXes of signed POLST forms are legal and valid. A copy should be retained in patient's medical record, on Ultra Pink paper when possible.

Using POLST

- Any incomplete section of POLST implies full treatment for that section.

Section A:

- If found pulseless and not breathing, no defibrillator (including automated external defibrillators) or chest compressions should be used on a person who has chosen "Do Not Attempt Resuscitation."

Section B:

- When comfort cannot be achieved in the current setting, the person, including someone with "Comfort Measures Only," should be transferred to a setting able to provide comfort (e.g., treatment of a hip fracture).
- Non-invasive positive airway pressure includes continuous positive airway pressure (CPAP), bi-level positive airway pressure (BiPAP), and bag valve mask (BVM) assisted respirations.
- IV antibiotics and hydration generally are not "Comfort Measures."
- Treatment of dehydration prolongs life. If person desires IV fluids, indicate "Limited Interventions" or "Full Treatment."
- Depending on local EMS protocol, "Additional Orders" written in Section B may not be implemented by EMS personnel.

Reviewing POLST

It is recommended that POLST be reviewed periodically. Review is recommended when:

- The person is transferred from one care setting or care level to another, or
- There is a substantial change in the person's health status, or
- The person's treatment preferences change.

Modifying and Voiding POLST

- A patient with capacity can, at any time, request alternative treatment.
- A patient with capacity can, at any time, revoke a POLST by any means that indicates intent to revoke. It is recommended that revocation be documented by drawing a line through Sections A through D, writing "VOID" in large letters, and signing and dating this line.
- A legally recognized decisionmaker may request to modify the orders, in collaboration with the physician, based on the known desires of the individual or, if unknown, the individual's best interests.

This form is approved by the California Emergency Medical Services Authority in cooperation with the statewide POLST Task Force. For more information or a copy of the form, visit **www.caPOLST.org**.

SEND FORM WITH PERSON WHENEVER TRANSFERRED OR DISCHARGED

35358373R00110

Made in the USA
Charleston, SC
06 November 2014